Christina Adams has a powerful, passionate, and convincing story to tell. Myself, I was looking for a camel milk source by page 38."
— RANDY FERTEL, PHD, author of *The Gorilla Man and the Empress of Steak* and cofounder of the Edible Schoolyard, New Orleans

"Christina Adams's writing and work are important to many indigenous cultures around the world, like my own nomadic tribe, the Tuareg camel herders. We need protecting."
— SIDI AMAR, nomad, camel handler, and Tuareg cultural protector, Sahara Desert, Niger

"If you think you know everything, then you haven't read Christina Adams's page-turning memoir about her quest for camel milk to help her son's autism. It's part the story of one mother's determination to help her son and part travel narrative, plus much camel lore. Adams has woven an incredible tapestry that will fascinate you with its science and touch you with its story. Reminiscent of John Vaillant's wonderful nonfiction book *The Tiger*, *Camel Crazy* will teach you things you never imagined and move you to tears."
— MARY MORRIS, author of *Gateway to the Moon* and *All the Way to the Tigers* (forthcoming)

"Christina Adams sweeps up the reader on her colorful, entertaining, and very personal quest to find out more about camels — and the exotic milk that proved so beneficial for her son and other autistic children. Her wonderful book takes us on fascinating travels, encounters, and discoveries, winding up with a useful trove of practical advice in the Appendix."
— NANCY JONES ABEIDERRAHMANE, founder of Tiviski and winner of the ROLEX Award for Enterprise

"In her fascinating book *Camel Crazy*, Christina Adams describes her quest to help her son, which is both heroic and an important reminder of the arrogance embedded in the prevailing wisdom of Western medicine and modern industrial life. We recklessly toss out important traditional knowledge, remove direct contact with the animals — like camels — who have shaped human civilization, and belittle the important steps to regain control over our lives by searching for answers in unexpected places. *Camel Crazy* is a joy to read and should inspire those of us who feel powerless in the face of industrialized life. Biodiversity matters. Animals matter. And it matters to enter into a space in which we consider possibilities that otherwise would seem impossible."

— RICHARD McCARTHY, executive director
of Slow Food International

"This brave, inspiring, and deeply exciting narrative is about Christina Adams's search for help for her son, which she found in the most unlikely of places — the milk of camels. She is the best kind of tour guide, propelling her intimate narrative through the Middle East to Amish country to a Manhattan doctor, and Adams does it all with such an infectious sense of wonder, a love of facts, and an insistence to get at the truth that I'd follow her anywhere. As she falls more and more in love with camels, so do we. This is a book that can change the world."

— CAROLINE LEAVITT, *New York Times* bestselling author of
Pictures of You and *Is This Tomorrow*

"*Camel Crazy* relates an extraordinary story and captures how camels represent freedom to pastoralists like me. This book's camel wisdom rings true and will help the humble animals who in turn sustain millions of pastoralists globally."

— ROBA B. JILO, camel herder and member of the
Karrayyu-Oromo tribe of Ethiopia

"As a self-professed 'beauty hunter,' I felt like I found the beauty-hunting bible within these pages. This is a book for anyone who believes in the power of belief, science, and love. Combining these things, Christina Adams has created a magical story that feels part memoir, part fairy tale, pure heart. I want everyone I know to read this book to be reminded how one woman can change the world by following her own path."

— JENNIFER PASTILOFF, bestselling author of *On Being Human:*
A Memoir of Waking Up, Living Real, and Listening Hard

"For me, as both a parent and self-advocate for autism spectrum disorder, seeing the development of science-based natural resources to increase functionality for people with autism is outstanding. Christina Adams has been an amazing international leader in finding solutions that geneticists are only now starting to understand. The trailblazing work she describes in this book has led to significant multidisciplinary scientific studies." — ANNE DELERY McWHORTER, autistic advocate and owner of Quiet Calm LLC

"A story as wondrous as a fantastic novel, full of amazing moments. This is an exploration fueled by love." — ANITA HUGHES, author of *California Summer: A Novel*

"Mesmerizing. Far more than an enchanting trip through camel lore and a look at the biology of this fascinating mammal, *Camel Crazy* offers a compelling description of how its milk quieted her young son's autism symptoms. Just as I was awaiting a scientific explanation, there it was, eloquent and exciting. Camels, and their milk, are indeed special." — RICKI LEWIS, PhD, author of *The Forever Fix: Gene Therapy and the Boy Who Saved It*

"Camel milk played, and continues to play, a huge role in our son Jack's nutrition. Our family is grateful to those like Christina Adams, who are forging a new path for those who need it most. Switching Jack to camel milk has been the single most beneficial thing we have done for our very picky eater." — THE HARRIS FAMILY, White Oak Pastures

"Combining a mother's love with the skill of a scientist and the finesse of a diplomatic ambassador, Christina Adams glides through international and cultural barriers with the realization that we are all part of a global village. In tirelessly striving to resolve her son's challenges, Adams expertly fits together several pieces of the puzzle in making fulfilling and productive lives for people on the autism spectrum more the rule rather than the exception." — STEPHEN M. SHORE, EdD, person with autism, author of *Beyond the Wall*, professor of special education at Adelphi University, and board member of Autism Speaks

CAMEL CRAZY

ALSO BY CHRISTINA ADAMS

A Real Boy: A True Story of Autism,
Early Intervention, and Recovery

CAMEL CRAZY

A Quest for Miracles in the Mysterious World of Camels

CHRISTINA ADAMS

Foreword by Joel Salatin

New World Library
Novato, California

New World Library
14 Pamaron Way
Novato, California 94949

The material in this book is intended for education. No expressed or implied guarantee
of the effects of the use of the recommendations can be given or liability taken. It is not
meant to take the place of diagnosis and treatment by a qualified medical practitioner or
therapist. Every effort has been made to confirm dates, names, and other aspects of the
episodes presented in this book and to use real names wherever possible, although a few
have been changed to protect privacy.

Text design by Tona Pearce Myers

Library of Congress Cataloging-in-Publication data is available.

First printing, October 2019
ISBN 978-1-60868-648-3
Ebook ISBN 978-1-60868-649-0
Printed in Canada on 100% postconsumer-waste recycled paper

New World Library is proud to be a Gold Certified Environmentally Responsible Publisher. Publisher certification awarded by Green Press Initiative.

10   9   8   7   6   5   4   3   2   1

To my beloved husband, our dear children,
and my exceptional mother

CONTENTS

Photographs follow page 172

Foreword by Joel Salatin   xiii

Introduction: Creeping Camelization   xvii

Chapter 1. Meeting the Camel   1

Chapter 2. The Next Step   4

Chapter 3. In a Camel No-Man's-Land   9

Chapter 4. Milk from Eden   14

Chapter 5. Project K: Where the Camels Are   18

Chapter 6. An Oasis of Camels   20

Chapter 7. Camel Milk Miracle   28

Chapter 8. The Milk Knows No Borders   35

Chapter 9. Camels: A God-Given Marvel?   40

Chapter 10. Forty-Eight Bottles of Milk in the Fridge   45

Chapter 11. Getting Close to Camels   47

Chapter 12. Healing with Camel Milk   53

Chapter 13. A Public Birth   59

Chapter 14. Camel Feel the Soul   68

Chapter 15. The Power of Camel Milk   73

Chapter 16. The Amish Take Camels on Faith   80

Chapter 17. A Camel Milk Savior   90

Chapter 18. A Fundamental Evolution   96

Chapter 19. You Knows Nothing about Camel   100

Chapter 20. Camel Farm Heaven   105

Chapter 21. Camel Milk in the Nobel Lab   120

Chapter 22. Doug Baum's World of Camels   128

Chapter 23. The Most Camel-Crazy Country in the World   134

Chapter 24. I Am a Camel Boy   140

Chapter 25. Marlin Takes a Stand   151

Chapter 26. Camel Clashes and Cultures   155

Chapter 27. What Kind of Crazy Thing Is Next?   160

Chapter 28. India Rediscovers Its Treasure   163

Chapter 29. An Old Camel Caste In the New India   170

Chapter 30. Help in Suffering   180

Chapter 31. Raika Village   186

Chapter 32. Raika Come In from the Cold (and I Collapse)   191

Chapter 33. Life in "The Sand"   200

Chapter 34. Camel Milk Seekers Have Questions   211

Chapter 35. Unto Her a Camel Is Born   214

Afterword: The World Wakes Up to Camels   217

Appendix: Camel Milk: A Users' Guide   222

Acknowledgments   242

Notes   245

Recommended Reading   254

Index   255

About the Author   267

FOREWORD

Few things tear at our heartstrings like a sick child. Sick old people, well, that just comes with the territory. But seeing a child suffer is among the darkest tragedies of the human experience. This amazing book tells how Christina Adams explored a hidden world to help her son, overcoming tremendous obstacles to create a miracle for children with autism. In doing so, she uncovers the incredible animal that helped create it.

Camel Crazy models all the nuances of a quest for truth. At the beginning, unbounded love motivates a search. The search yields solutions — a true success for mother, son, and then the world. But none of it was easy. How did she get to this point?

Things have changed in children's health — some for the better, some for the worse. My work with food has taught me a few things about that. Prior to the rise of industrial farming, processed junk food, and chemical agriculture, the common childhood illnesses — indeed, most human sicknesses — were infectious diseases such as pneumonia, whooping cough, measles, diphtheria, and gastroenteritis. Many of these arose from a lack of basic medicine and good sanitation.

Today, these diseases have largely been eliminated in developed countries, but other childhood illnesses are rising: diabetes, cancer — and autism. Our food supply, soil, air, water, and ways of living have turned toxic, and kids are paying the price. Research shows that many new cases of autism may be linked to environmental triggers (chemicals, pollution, the stuff of modern life). But help for kids with autism is hard to find. Sometimes it's downright impossible.

Because some of autism's symptoms aren't obvious, society can easily ignore it. But for people with autism and their caregivers, the condition can mean a lifelong tunnel of pain and expense, and can come with food intolerances, gastrointestinal issues, emotional challenges, loneliness, and the risk of an early death. I've learned from Dr. Temple Grandin, a brilliant livestock scientist with autism, that folks on the autism spectrum can excel at some valuable jobs. But they need the chance to develop their skills so they can live a full life.

In the US healthcare system, where all resources are tightly managed, there is little time for busy doctors to look into natural healing methods. They can offer expensive patented medications or lifestyle advice, which patients may or may not listen to. Doctors know that good health isn't only found in a lab or through medication. But it takes money to push health research through the sieve of regulations. And some kids need help that can't be found in a pill bottle or a therapy. This is when parents throw up their hands and say, If no one can help my child, what can I do?

This book is the story of a woman who has traveled the earth to find help for her child, and other children. She found a solution in the most unlikely of places. Without ever intending to, she became a leader in today's self-empowered health movement. She's bringing us knowledge about the medicinal value of traditional wisdom, earth-based living, and the forgotten gifts of nature. And she's educating doctors and moving science forward.

One narrative thread in *Camel Crazy* is Christina Adams's experience of dealing with the barriers of official resistance. Another is the joy of discovering the wonderful nature of the camel. The West has relegated this animal to television commercials and zoos, but in much of the world, the camel has been the backbone of life for millennia. What the bison are to Native Americans, camels are to countless people around the planet. Christina's portrait of the camel as loving and responsive, a companion as well as a working animal, is truly eye-opening.

As a livestock farmer, I identify deeply with her moving portraits of "camel whisperers" and the partnerships between animals and humans. Her celebration of the diversity of "cameleers" of Muslim, Jewish, Amish, and Hindu backgrounds adds to the depth and breadth of the narrative. The captured dialogues reveal how everyone pushes through language and religious differences to care for camels and help other people. These charming caretakers of the "ships of the desert" are precious stewards of knowledge, protecting their animals' great genetic legacy as they help preserve this planet. I know you will love them as much as I do, after hearing them share their secrets in these pages.

These are great reasons to read *Camel Crazy*. But the most important reason is the perseverance and determination of a loving mother seeking to care for her child. The book flows beautifully, perhaps because Christina does not pause to overanalyze her doubts or her encounters with potential naysayers, be they friends or government regulators. She focuses on the breakthroughs and moves the story along quickly, from hurdle to jump. Imagining how hard this was makes me ache with exhaustion. How could she keep going? Because she soldiered on for her child, then for others.

When I see mothers and fathers raising their children with haste, stopping for fast food, afraid to ask questions, refusing to consider a deeper and quite sensible approach to health, I want to stop them and ask: "Do you think? Do you care? Does it matter?"

Christina and this story are an inspiration for action and education. The book is a courageous trumpet call to seek innovative solutions and then lead, rather than simply accept and follow. Christina had an idea that few people would have thought of. She dared to seek where others would have quit. She communicated with people some would find intimidating. She pursued when others would have stopped. This is a book about love, truth, and survival, a story of courage and passion. We can all use a big dose of those.

— JOEL SALATIN, international lecturer, pioneering farmer, and author of twelve books, including *Holy Cows and Hog Heaven* and *Folks, This Ain't Normal* (www.polyfacefarms.com)

INTRODUCTION

Creeping Camelization

Before camels entered my life, I rarely gave them a thought. They seemed like relics of history, marooned in time amid palm trees and pyramids. But when I met a camel in suburban California, I suddenly realized that its milk might help my son. Only instinct drove me to find it. Back then there was no online information, no expert or book to consult about the sources or benefits of camel milk. Little was known about camels outside (or sometimes even inside) the countries they've inhabited for eons.

As camels became part of my life, I grew entranced by them and their keepers, whose stories glittered like potsherds in sand. As my camel friends piled up, so did the gifts they offered. I have statues, photographs, bracelets carved from bone. Farmers tossed me camel baseball caps, veterinarians gave me scarves. I have a camel T-shirt from Dubai and a silver camel necklace from Israel or Palestine, depending on who you ask.

In the house where I write today, three tiny jeweled camels prance across my desk. My kitchen shelf holds a chocolate camel wrapped in gold foil, from Dubai. He guards camel milk powder in bottles and sky-blue packets, bagged industrial samples and beribboned Indian chocolates. There are energy drinks labeled in purple Arabic script. My refrigerator holds raw and pasteurized milk, colostrum, and kefir, a cultured milk that I hate but nomads and health fanatics love. My cellphone, on the dining table, holds a photo of camel-hump fat. The only camel items I don't have, besides meat, are cheese (it's hard to make) and urine — and if I was terribly sick, I might try that too.

I am not a crazy camel lady. I don't have a camel farm. But I am camel crazy. It's a natural consequence of seeing those bottles of precious milk work a miracle in my son. As a writer and researcher, I'm compelled to tell our story, and the wonders of this amazing animal.

Until now, the secrets of ancient camel peoples have been preserved mostly in oral legend. In India today, camel keepers still stand on one leg each morning as they balance a pot on their other knee, milking the teat of a she-camel into a foamy bowl. They drink it along with a mildly narcotic tea to start their day. But camels are mainly seen as curiosities, roadside tourist attractions, zoo animals, the toothy cartoon on a cigarette packet. Even the great camel cultures of the Middle East have mostly lost their knowledge of the milk's restorative power.

Yet camels, like their image as a symbol of the desert, are hard to kill. Once the main transport of the great Silk Road trade routes that formed modern civilization, they still carry salt blocks, trucks, and entire households on their backs. They've never truly disappeared from the wadis, dunes, steppes, and forests where they evolved and were domesticated.

My immersion in camel cultures enriched my understanding of the health properties of the milk. I first focused on its benefits for children with autism, but even the scanty science, along with traditional lore, suggested that it held promise for other health conditions as well. Those years of close attention gave me a unique depth of knowledge. But just as enriching has been my love for the animals and their keepers.

As one Pakistani camel friend says, "Camel feel the soul." This quiet, devoted, wary, intensely loyal, vociferous, blubbering, delicate, gossipy, sociable, cliquish, powerful, mysterious, and extraordinarily gifted beast provokes passion. Its admirers are just as intense as the animals, probably more so.

And now the global herd of camels (estimated at thirty-five million, up from twenty million during my first year of research) and camel lovers is growing. The modern demand for camel milk and meat is bringing camels to farms and towns all over. It will inevitably rise in parallel with increasing rates of autism (which now affects an estimated 2 to 3 percent of children worldwide), food allergies, diabetes, and other disorders. Camels are being used to treat snakebite and in cancer research, among other innovations. Their bodies are preadapted for high temperatures and droughts, making them the perfect animal for the world's changing climate. Yet even in societies that have traditionally tended camels, they're a well-kept secret today.

So yes, I'm camel crazy. And I'm not alone. We are myriad. Determined. And maybe you will join the herd.

NOTE

In creating this book, I've written dialogue the way it was spoken or written by the speakers (for whom English is often a second, third, or fourth language). My aim is to convey their thoughts without imposing someone else's interpretation. The spelling of names and terms from other cultures follows the usage of my sources. I've worked to clarify customs, faiths, and narrative lenses by consulting with the people who live them. This is truly a group endeavor, and I am grateful to everyone who chose to share their stories.

1   MEETING THE CAMEL

"What else do they do with the milk?"

— ME TO A CAMEL MAN

The camel stands calmly, munching something hay-like, placid in her dirty-blond summer coat. Her great head grows like a question mark from the curve of her muscular neck. Padded leathery feet keep her comfortable on the bare spots of the lawn. She ignores the children offering pink tufts of cotton candy, staring at her with freckles ringing the Os of their open mouths. She was trundled in a horse van to this college in Orange County, California, two hours and a rocky mountain from her home in fire-scorched farm country. Her eyes watch the humans scattered on the green grass at this Sunday afternoon book festival. Her long lashes hide the clear inner eyelid that will automatically close if an unlikely coastal sandstorm roars in.

    This camel knows her mission. She tolerates the admiring glances and rude remarks, like "What's a *camel* doing here?" She knows that her human owner, the alpha bull of her herd, is nearby if she needs him. Little can faze her, as she has no natural predators and a nuanced startle reflex, although fluttering fabric and sudden movements may annoy her. Her eyes express a confident view of her place in the world, composed at this moment of a task, the pen that holds her, and something to nibble, with a little water on the side. Today, her job is to be a camel at a fair.

What she doesn't know is that her blood can work medical miracles, her flesh is kin to that of million-dollar racing camels, her organs are debated, and her milk has healed the sick for centuries. She also doesn't know that she's about to launch a movement that will drive her species's price sky-high, that people will clamor for the milk she gives, which will help fuel a modern resurgence of her kind.

Neither do I. At this moment, she's just a camel, and I'm just a fearful, newly separated single mother. She will inspire me to seek the surprising remedy for my son's autism symptoms, and to become a camel milk expert. This creature will throw me into research, dispatch me across the United States, India, and the United Arab Emirates, and send my words to places like Malaysia, Sweden, England, Cyprus, Mongolia, France, and Pakistan. She'll cause scoffing and admiration, inspire scientific research and many products.

But now I stand by her broad side, as bored as she is, watching her. She's tall and stolid, seemingly unflappable. Camels are like that, able to keep going without complaint for miles and kilometers, hauling salt, fat-bellied tourists, large milk cans, towing wagons, trucks, and carts draped in glittering scarlet curtains, carrying entire households on their backs. But I don't know this. I just wonder why a camel's here if none of these kids are riding it.

I see the long eyelashes blink once. I spot a flapping tent behind her and walk over to investigate. There are small white bottles of camel milk lotion. And soaps. I like soap. I lift a smooth, wavy bar to smell it, and the scent of lavender moves lightly across my upper lip. A man in a green baseball cap shifts behind the counter. "Hi," I say. "Is that your camel?"

"Yes, sure is. We make soap and lotions from camel milk. Very natural and healthy stuff."

I try a dab of the white lotion. It's thin and spreads easily, as light as sunshine. Then I ask, "What else do they do with the milk?"

I don't know why I'm asking. Perhaps boredom is driving me to prolong the chat, or maybe it's just how I am, always curious. Probably both.

"They give it to premature babies in hospitals in the Middle East. It's supposed to not cause any allergies."

"Really? It's nonallergenic milk?"

"It's said to be close to mother's milk, like breast milk."

"Thanks."

I look at my son, Jonah, sitting on a nearby slope, knees nestled in the grass as he reads an airplane book. His four years of autism therapies have cost half a million dollars. Right now he's a happy, blue-eyed, seven-year-old charmer fitting few people's idea of autism, but a trace amount of milk can send him into a trance, staring at a wall or laughing at nothing. He can disappear inside his head or up a ladder, atop a wall or anywhere. Or one day, I worry, out of his classroom and into special ed.

I bring my son to the camel, stand him before the rounded belly and single hump. I tell him, "It's a camel," and he says, "Okay, Mom."

I have to find this milk.

2 THE NEXT STEP

"My people love the camels."
— ELHADJI KOUMAMA

Back home from the fair in the house of my expiring marriage, I steal a few minutes in my office, tapping at my keyboard as Jonah watches television. Research isn't new to me — it has slowly become my life. No child passes a kindergarten readiness test with autism undetected without a parent who does the work. He's had behavioral, speech, occupational, and social skills therapies, medications and supplements, plus coaching from me around the clock. It's a boon that I started my now-vanished career at the Pentagon. Working in politics, aerospace, and public relations has taught me how to figure things out. But living the therapy lifestyle has provided a whole new education. Studying psychology, biology, law, and medicine has quickened my intuition.

While holding that sweet-smelling bar of camel milk soap, I'd had two ideas. One: If they give camel milk to premature babies, maybe it could reboot Jonah's immune system, the way human breast milk enriches an infant's health. That might stabilize his functioning, which goes haywire not only on milk and cheese, but on sugar and other carbohydrates as well. I've seen the changes reflected in his lab tests. Maybe we could get smoother conversation, as he needs to develop more social skills to accompany his perfect enunciation. Maybe it could

4

help him live more easily in the world. Two: This would be a great dairy substitute for people who can't drink regular milk. I could make his cupcakes and a hundred other foods with this milk!

My computer search for "camel milk" reveals four, maybe five PubMed citations. These items, from an international database of medical journal articles, read like a foreign language. The articles I click on are obscure reports from remote countries. There's something about failed attempts to make cheese and a slightly revolting paper about wound healing. But that's it. I print out the pages and stack them neatly on my desk. As I go to make his dinner, I look longingly back, and promise myself that I won't forget.

A couple of months later, on a rainy New Year's Day, we have to leave the lovely home where Jonah was raised. His father, who still lives there, is keeping the house. When we sat down to tell Jonah we were divorcing, our son said, "You guys have spent a lot of time apart, and you argue a lot. Will I live in a house with a second story?"

"Yes," I said. I knew he wanted an upstairs.

"Yay!" he said, raising his arms in the air. "A second story, just what I always wanted!" But then he sobered. "So I'll visit Dad, but you'll still take care of me mainly, right?" He looked at me for reassurance, but he wasn't really upset.

"Yes," I said, hiding my tears with great relief. After everything we had been through, I admired him so much. I couldn't prevent this home from crumbling, but at least he would be happy about the new place I'd had to fight for.

Now we live in a two-story condominium behind a freeway and a convenience store, near other stores offering massages and payday loans. Child and spousal support from Jonah's father will temporarily keep us afloat. I have fantasies of moving to New York as I'm traveling to speak on autism and my new book. But as I am Jonah's primary caregiver, with less help than before, my writing's always cut short.

To make money, I try freelance business writing. But I can hear Jonah jumping off the sofa or kicking the upstairs balcony he's hanging from as I interview executives by phone (I give up). School meetings, cooking foods for his special diet, pharmacy visits, blood draws, brain scans, and six-hour round trips to his doctor take up my time. There are play dates, after-school lessons, his homework and mine (for the divorce). His busy hands constantly investigate and break things apart. Sometimes he intelligently talks me to death. When we're out for a casual dinner, I grab and hide parts of his bread, rice, and limp cheese-free pizza to keep his carbohydrate load down. More than a small serving can send him into overdrive, making him wild, silly, and unreachable. Doses of digestive enzymes help a little, until the company changes the formula. I subsist on handfuls of nuts and grow thin and isolated. My main relief is visiting the gym, slamming balls in an echoing squash court.

Every morning, I grind Jonah's medicines into a sippy cup and mix up his potato milk, a powdery substitute for the cow, goat, and rice milks he can't tolerate. (Nut milks cause allergic reactions, and soy contains estrogens that may not be good for young boys.) Every afternoon, I monitor his after-school snacks for traces of dairy. But I don't forget about camel milk. One day while Jonah is at school, I drive to the library of the University of California, Irvine. Scrolling through PubMed again, I find a small trove of camel citations. Camel diseases, camel diets, camel mastitis, camel — wait.

"Etiology of Autism and Camel Milk as Therapy." It's a brief new article, published a few months ago by the Israeli veterinarian Reuven Yagil and another researcher, Yosef Shabo. When children with autism were given camel milk, their symptoms improved, although the study only covers short-term results. There's another study by the same authors: "Camel Milk for Food Allergies in Children." It says that eight children recovered from severe food allergies, mainly to milk, by using camel milk as a treatment of "last resort." So somebody else has thought about this too!

We're under attack from cheese. It makes my son flap his hands and walk on tiptoe (a sign of neurological disorders), pace in circles, and detach: it makes him act "autistic." He doesn't do these things on a dairy-free regimen. Although I ban dairy from his diet, it turns up everywhere. If camel milk can help with food reactions, it's a far better remedy than I'd hoped.

I go home and keep reading about camels, about the countries where they live: Saudi Arabia, Kuwait, Ethiopia, Pakistan, Kenya. I find an online list of camels for sale in America, but no one writes me back.

At the gym, I tell Bash, a new squash- and polo-playing acquaintance, about my camel milk hunt. A thirty-something entrepreneur from Pakistan, Bash says he's heard of camels in Israel. He offers to bring some milk back from his next business trip there. He treats Jonah and me to a horse-riding lesson, and we canter against the blue California sky, my worries briefly vanishing in laughter. Sometimes there is kindness in the world.

In early summer, I attend a jewelry party at a well-to-do friend's house. But this isn't your typical suburban jewelry show. A nearly seven-foot-tall man called Elhadji Koumama is showcasing his jewelry and leather goods. Majestic in a tobacco-brown robe and purple-black head wrap, he places a thin silver bracelet on my wrist. It's engraved and has a raised edge. His family made it. "We call that style camel-back."

"You have camels in your country?" I ask.

"Do we have camels? Oh, in Niger, we have so many camels. My people love the camels. We take them very far in the desert, making a caravan. Bringing salt. You never heard of that?"

"I've heard of Niger, but not the camel part. Where is it?"

He smiles warmly, revealing strong teeth. "It's very far away from here. You can come visit. But don't come now. The rain is very bad and the wind too strong, too many sandstorms. Wait till the weather is better."

He is a Tuareg, a member of a tribe that lives in and around the Sahara Desert. "Sure, we drink the camel milk all the time. You come, you will drink it, stay with my family."

I didn't even know how to say the name of his country properly, but I know it's in Africa. He pronounces it *Nee-jair*, with a French *j*, like *je suis*, meaning "I am." And *je suis* curious about him, because he knows camels. For hundreds of years, his people have traveled with them. "Do you think any of your people would come over here and take care of camels? Sell the milk?"

He smiles. "No, I don't think they want to leave where they are. Maybe they could come and help for a little while, but not stay." To hear someone casually reject the American lifestyle makes me wonder what allure the alternative holds. It must be pretty good over there for these devoted camel people. The desert of Niger sounds very far away, but I like the idea of a place that has sandstorms and camels.

I buy the camelback bracelet. Elhadji gives me blessings and good wishes. The host takes a photo. Later when I look at it, I see my arms bare against his sleeve. Only his face shows outside his garments. We are both smiling.

3 IN A CAMEL NO-MAN'S-LAND

"Battling thousands of years of tradition isn't easy."
— Dr. Amnon Gonenne

It's nearing Christmas when my friend Bash goes to Israel. I'm at a chilly outdoor café when he calls me on his return. "You want the good news or the bad first?"

"Bad first."

"Okay. First, I got some milk. It wasn't as easy as I thought," he said. "We had to drive pretty far to get it. I had a friend to help. I actually got it on the plane."

"Great!"

"But when I got to JFK in New York, they wouldn't let it in. Customs threw it away."

"Oh no!"

"But wait," he says. "I think you can do this, but it has to be the right way. I found a guy you can call in Israel. Plus, with me being Pakistani, and Muslim, maybe it's best that I not travel with any suspicious packages, you know?" he says wryly. I hadn't thought of that. How sad that a person carrying out a good deed has to bear the added weight of racial profiling. But he gives me a number. "Somebody smart, a doctor or professor, who knows about camel milk," he says.

At home alone in a quiet house, I take a deep breath and call Israel.

The foreign ringtone heightens my suspense. A man answers gruffly, not in English.

"I'm calling from the US. I got your number from a friend. I'm looking for camel milk."

"Oh. I was asleep." It's around 11:30 p.m., he says. Luckily he speaks enough English to tell me "Call this man" and give me another number. I apologize deeply. He isn't too happy but is still very helpful. I feel guilty — but now I have a connection. I fall on the bed, staring delightedly at the ceiling.

Next day, I realize I know nothing about Israel. Images of Bible scenes and dancing the hora come to me. Falafel. The Palestinian strife and the bombing of outdoor cafés, where I vow never to sit if I go there. I know about World War II and Jewish homeland history. But modern Israel seems like a polished place, so the fact that they even have camels is surprising.

I call the number I was given. The man who answers is Eyal, and he's apparently the owner of a camel farm. "Yes, I have camel milk," he says. His English is very limited.

"I want to ask you some questions about the milk. How do you test it? Has anyone used it for health reasons?"

We stumble over words. He makes a fast decision. "My uncle, he's doctor. He can talk to you." He gives me another number. Soon I'm speaking to a deep voice with no trace of an Israeli accent.

From Tel Aviv, Dr. Amnon Gonenne says, "Hello. I know some things about camel milk. What do you want to know?" He's an informal adviser to Eyal, sort of a family member if not an uncle by blood.

"Are you an MD?"

"I'm a PhD and researcher. I work in biological sciences. Cancer is my most recent focus," he says concisely. This is how Amnon says everything, I'll come to know. Trained at Israeli and California institutions, he's got a brilliant scientific mind. The most remarkable part is its openness, a quality many doctors tend to lose.

"I have a feeling camel milk might help my son. So I'm trying to find it."

"Why? Does he have cancer or a disease?"

"No, thankfully. He has autism. I heard the milk is nonallergenic," I say. "And I hope it can help his immune system."

"Why would he need that? What kind of conditions does he have, in addition to autism?" He hasn't heard of the new Israeli publication.

"Some kids with autism have a very impaired immune system. He's on medications for it. Also, he can't handle cow milk, and sugars and other carbs make him hyperactive and silly." His silence tells me this is a new concept to him. I try again.

"Autism is classified by the DSM as a developmental or psychological disorder, and thought to be untreatable," I explain. I outline the basic description: a cluster of symptoms including narrow interests, social problems, and repetitive behaviors. I say how these are often accompanied by digestive and immune-system issues. Genes are part of the picture. In addition, environmental factors like pollution, power sources, pesticides and other chemicals, and parental exposure to toxins can alter genetic expression. While identification of previously unrecognized autism cases accounts for some of the increase, the fast-rising American autism rate is real and continues apace. In short, autism is a mystery, just like camel milk.

"But really," I add, "when the kids' other health symptoms are treated, they can get much better."

"So tell me what you want to know," he says. "Do you have Skype?"

A day later, there he is on my screen, a serious, brown-eyed man with olive skin, graying hair, and an analytic manner, sitting at a desk in his study. He only sees me once: my computer camera fails and I can't get it to work. But every few days, it's his face and my voice, exchanging studies and conjecturing about camel milk, inflammation, autism, and disease.

"In some kids, autism comes with extreme food sensitivities. I track my son's diet and allergic response in his blood work, and it matches his behavior." I tell him about the rise and fall of my son's eosinophil levels, the white blood cells that fight infection and mediate allergic response. He explains that inflammation is connected to certain health conditions, including cancer and bowel diseases. I watch his thick black brows move slightly, his fingers pressed in a triangle as he speaks.

Having grown up in Israel after his family fled the Holocaust, Amnon is familiar with camels. He drinks camel milk every day, plus a quarter cup of high-quality olive oil. "Olive oil has a protective effect on the liver," he says. There are only three known inflammation fighters, he states, other than some immunosuppressant drugs: steroids, aspirin, and olive oil. "And now I think camel milk may be one," he adds. In Israel, the main users of Eyal's milk are men with Crohn's disease (an inflammatory bowel condition), who are drinking one eight-ounce cup (236 milliliters) of camel milk a day and improving quite a bit. The milk they drink is raw, not pasteurized.

"Where does the milk come from?" I ask him.

"It comes from the Negev Desert. Bedouins keep the camels, and the milk comes from them."

Eyal has a clever arrangement with the nomadic herders. He leases their camels in the spring, when the babies are born. Female camels give milk only when their babies are with them, and not much at that: just four to five liters a day, about one-eighth of what cows produce. Around eight to ten months later, they are impregnated again and stop giving milk. They return to the Bedouins to graze on desert vegetation for up to sixteen months. "That's a long pregnancy, poor things!" I say.

"It's usually around thirteen months, give or take, which also limits the supply," says Amnon. "Some of the plants may add medicinal value to the milk, but we don't know for sure." Once the babies are born, Eyal takes the camels back and starts milking them again.

Some customers pick the milk up from Eyal; for others he delivers it, like an old-fashioned milkman. But it's not a typical business. One night we're about to chat when Amnon says, "Hold, please." I sit at my desk as the minutes pass. Finally he reappears. "Sorry. I was on the line with a hospital."

"Is everything okay?"

"Yes. A patient is about to have surgery, and they want to give camel milk to fortify her. I had to give information to the rabbi and the doctor. It's fine now."

"So they're going to give it to her?"

"Yes. I just had to help them approve the process. Camel milk isn't officially legal in Israel."

"Why not?"

"It's not allowed in the Jewish religion. The camel is considered to have a split hoof, which means it is forbidden for food, although it actually has a soft, two-toed foot, not a hoof. It's a very clean animal, remarkably so. But battling thousands of years of tradition isn't easy."

"So how do people get to drink the milk?"

"You can get permission from a rabbi, but it has to be for a sickness that can't be sufficiently treated any other way. It helps to say that you don't like the taste. And you certainly can't let on that you enjoy it."

So camel milk operates on the fringe. A social, legal no-man's-land. But if it turns out to be good for my son, I couldn't care less.

4 MILK FROM EDEN

"Nobody really does it, but you did."
— Eyal

A few weeks later, in my bedroom upstairs, I'm online with Amnon again. "Christina, do you still want the milk?"

"Yes, of course, Amnon," I say.

"You feel that you have enough information, and this is what you want to do?"

I'm surprised that after all this time, he's still asking. Maybe he's making sure I'm consenting.

"Nothing is without risk, but the risk seems minimal," I say. "Is there anything else I should know?"

"I agree. And no, not that I am aware of."

"Milk will be arriving from Israel, in the Los Angeles area," he says carefully, after a pause. "I am not sure how much there will be."

One of Amnon's sons is an American MD. His little daughter has severe irritable bowel disease, and Amnon wants her to try the milk. Now he's sending some with a person I don't know.

A few days pass. I hold off on making plans for the weekend, but nothing happens.

Then he calls. "An Israeli family is returning to their Los Angeles home." Their four-year-old bleeds terribly from his bowels. The child is developmentally normal in every way, but no doctor can solve this

14

problem. The family heard about camel milk while in Israel. "They just returned, and they got it past customs. Can you go get the bottles and share some with my granddaughter? Hopefully there should be enough for your son, but I'm not sure yet."

I drive an hour up the freeway and park outside a stucco house, not far from some Orthodox Jewish neighborhoods. I knock, and the boy's father brings out some tall one-liter bottles that I slip quickly into a cooler.

In wonder that I have camel milk in my back seat, I navigate the dark sea of freeway taillights as carefully as if there's a beating heart in the cooler. At home, I slide the frozen bottles sideways into the freezer compartment of my refrigerator and go upstairs to sleep. It seems amazing to me in my king-size bed, watching a tiny red light shining from my alarm clock, that foreign bottles lie undisturbed downstairs, like a sunken treasure beneath a questing ship.

The next afternoon I stand outside under a small green tree. The sky soars a perfect blue above the sidewalk. Holding the bottle of frozen camel milk feels like a leap across time and space. Images of faceless Bedouins wrapped in desert clothes come to me, a great space arching between us. Soon I'll pick Jonah up from school, and he'll throw his arms around my neck and squeeze too hard, run into the house and turn on a cartoon, and jump with glee on the sofa. I'm so happy. I have camel milk at last.

Amnon calls. "Did you receive the milk?"

"Yes, I did."

"Good condition?"

"Perfect."

I split the shipment according to his instructions and send half to Amnon's son up north, packed in dry ice. The bottles arrive in fine shape. But now I seek more for Jonah. A few bottles won't be enough for a longer trial. Some medications and diets cause changes overnight, others take a month to figure out. There's something important about this milk, and I don't even question what I'm doing. In a few more weeks, I get my big chance.

"The flight will arrive in the evening. Meet the mother at the gate," instructs Amnon. Because I'm not sure it's legal to bring raw "exotic" milk into the United States but don't want to ask, I'm a little tense, but I'm going full speed ahead. I've obtained a medical letter explaining why the milk is an appropriate treatment for Jonah. As day turns to dusk, I race to Los Angeles Airport to wait for the mother arriving on the El Al flight. Will the milk make it here unspoiled? The bottles have been in the aircraft hold for the fifteen hours, plus transit time to the airport. Just one airport worker getting bossy or careless could ruin our plan. The milk could be confiscated or melted into a puddle.

Time passes, maybe an hour. She knows I'm a five-foot-seven, blue-eyed blonde wearing red. But no one comes through the door. The plane has landed. What's the problem? As another half hour passes, I grow nervous. Have they stopped her? Taken the milk? "What's taking so long?" I ask someone.

"It's customs, it always takes at least an hour." I feel stupid and kind of embarrassed — having traveled only twice internationally in the past ten years, I've forgotten. Much later, frazzled passengers appear, hugging people as they stream out, speaking a language I don't recognize. Still, there's no woman fitting the description I've been given, and people stop coming. Did I get the flight number wrong? I'm starting to panic. Then the door opens slowly for a dark-haired woman with two kids and a stack of luggage. She looks at me and smiles tiredly.

After hoisting the navy suitcase into the trunk of my Volvo, I unzip it and stare at the contents. Twenty-four bottles lie side by side in a Styrofoam case, lined up like iceberg soldiers. I roll down the freeway, bringing my prize to safety.

The next day my cell rings while I'm outside. It's Eyal. "Did you get the milk?"

"Yes, it's fine."

"It is cold?"

"Frozen like a rock."

"Christina."

"Yes?"

"Please I say something to you. Is okay?"

"Okay, sure."

"Many people say they would go all over the world to help their child," he says. His English is hesitant with emotion. "But to see a mother who did it? Nobody really does it, but you did."

His solemn recognition startles me, touches a soft spot in my heart. He makes me feel like someone, in this hard and lonely world.

5 PROJECT K

Where the Camels Are

"Just get down there!"

— COLLEGE STUDENTS

At first, I don't think of camels themselves, just their milk. In the rare moments when I actually think of the animals, I imagine cardboard cutouts you'd shuffle across a game board. They don't seem particularly special to me. But I wish I could fly a herd in. The world is supposed to have around twenty million camels. Why can't I have a few?

As I puzzle over the best way to give camel milk to Jonah and monitor the results, Amnon and I chat about Kazakhstan, a country I have to look for on a map. He says it has lots of camels, and they're cheap. To compare, I look at Australia, where they're killing unwanted camels. A pregnant Aussie camel costs ten thousand dollars (people buy them pregnant to ensure they can breed). You can fly them in on a 747 cargo plane. It sounds ludicrous, but someone actually did it. Boats are out, as lengthy sea travel isn't good for them. I imagine tall, goofy cartoon camels in little sailor hats on deck, craning their necks wistfully toward land.

I serve as a guest speaker for a business class at Chapman University. The teacher asks the students to analyze my ideas and develop a project on camel milk production. The undergrads are intrigued with Project K, as we call it (for Kazakhstan, the home of all those cheap camels). I divide the students into groups to make business plans. When presentation day comes, two of the three groups surprise me with the same recommendation.

"There's a camel farm not far from here, near San Diego. You should go see if they'll start a dairy. It's too hard to bring camels from outside, or to do it in Kazakhstan and bring the milk here."

"What's the name of it?"

"Oasis Camel Dairy."

"But they don't sell milk, do they?" I ask.

"Call them, or just get down there!" The students are more excited over Project K than I expected, smiling and debating each other. They even present me with a mock-up of a camel milk carton.

I follow their recommendation and call the Oasis Camel Dairy, explaining that I'm looking for camel milk because I think it might help my son and be a great dairy substitute. I ask whether they have ever thought about selling milk.

The man on the other end of the line has never heard of camel milk helping autism. But he says, "We've had a few calls lately from people interested in buying the place."

"Really? From where?"

"All over. So we'd really decided not to meet anyone else. We just don't have the time."

How can I convince him I'm not just one of the herd?

"I guess for me, I'm not doing it for a big commercial thing. I'm doing it as a mother, because it can help so many people. So if you just want to talk a little, I won't stay long."

"Okay, I think we can do that."

Whew. I'm heading into the camel unknown.

6 AN OASIS OF CAMELS

"I have a way."

— CAMEL HANDLER GIL RIEGLER

The waves splash the coastline as I drive south on Pacific Coast Highway. I'm in boots because I don't know if a camel farm is a big industrial place or a muddy lot. It's January, and the wind tears at my windshield as I merge left onto I-5. I pass the white, breast-like domes of a nuclear plant, speed through immigration checkpoints with caution signs depicting a running woman and child. A desolate marine base and a naval warfare station occupy the stark brown hills for miles. At Oceanside, I turn inland. The suburbs roll by, and then the harsh winter sun reveals an exurban desert. The road winds up into a rugged little Switzerland, through mountains littered with white stones, then down through skeletal trees burned black by wildfires. A bright-orange spray-painted sign reads "Ostrich eggs for sale." Small wineries and little houses with rusty swing sets flash by. Horse trailers lean over weedy ditches.

A feedstore marks the entrance to Ramona, a dusty farm town with Mexican restaurants, antique shops, and a couple of drinkers' bars. Leaving Ramona, I enter a cloud-swept agrarian valley with a giant egg farm. But now I'm lost. I drive partway back to Ramona, then pull over and call. Back I go.

A tiny sign reading "Oasis Camel Dairy" sits high on a post of galvanized plumbing pipe. I get out and open the gate, then chain it again behind me; I spent my teens on a farm, and farm memory never dies. The tires crunch with a familiar sound over the gravel path. When I park, a black-and-white dog runs up and plants its feet in my lap.

Outside the weathered red farmhouse, a raft of speckled turkeys gobbles in unison in a pen, their wings fanning as they move, like wind passing over a wheat field. There's a small donkey by a bush, silent as a statue. A dark-haired man in a plaid farmer's jacket comes out. "Hi, you made it," he says. "I'm Gil. Come upstairs." I follow him up the outside steps and walk almost straight into their kitchen table.

Like most farmhouses, the place looks rigged more for function than style, with a well-used birdcage right by the door. Beyond the kitchen is a cozy living room, but instead of graduation photos or religious portraits on the walls, the icons seem to be camels. Through the dust-soft daylight I spot camel statues and dull-bright woven beaded fabrics made by foreign hands.

"Would you like to go see the camels?" Gil asks politely.

"Sure, yes, if it's not too much trouble."

We walk through the backyard into the fenced-off pasture. Tufts of yellow-green winter grass crest like whitecaps in a sea of brown dirt. Islands of gray rocks rise in the distance. I spot a tall sand-brown camel whose hump looms larger and larger as we approach, blocking out the weak sun.

"This is Camelot. Hi, boy," says Gil, scratching the camel's head. Gil cups his face and smooches Camelot's long white nose. The camel stands stock-still. I hang back, searching my mind for something comparable, and come up with *horse*. But the legs are much longer, the barrel stomach rises into the hump like a volcano, and those floppy feet could never wear horseshoes. Two steps closer, I see whiskers poking from grayish lips. A curly topknot sits between the ears, and blond tufts edge the tawny jawline. The camel doesn't seem displeased, but his long-lashed amber eyes don't deign to notice me. He gazes forward, his arched head like a Roman centurion in a helmet. Gil strokes him and soothingly murmurs, "Yes, good boy, how you doin'?"

Gil turns to me, his green eyes steady and calm. "You can touch him." I put my arm out. The camel's neck is so high that I have to stretch to reach his forehead. His face is gentle geometry, a sloping rectangle with slit nostrils, capped by diamond-shaped ears. My fingers touch his knotty crown. He shifts his head slightly. "He's a great camel, but may not be in the best mood today," Gil says.

We walk toward another. "This is Goldie," he says. With two slender white front legs, she looks more feminine than Camelot, the color of light honey. Her wind-tossed blond fur is tucked behind her ears.

"Her father was pure white, and mom was brown. Goldie's really a devoted camel. She gives me milk."

"Don't they all give milk?"

"It's hard to get camels to give their milk, so that's one of the problems with milking them on a bigger scale. They need the baby to stimulate them to produce milk. But she does it for me."

Before I can ask how, I spot a narrow little camel with matchstick legs.

"And here's her baby boy," says Gil, his soft voice filling with pride. The calf is cookie-colored, with soft, curly brown hair and a hump tipped with black. His spindly forelegs kick out like he's surprised, and he bounces on the grassy dirt, leaping back and forth like a rocking horse. Goldie stands impassively, as many mothers do, while he gambols in the sparse hay of the shed.

"And what's that one?"

Taller than Camelot and Goldie, this camel is slim but has a very wide chest. We walk over, but Gil cautions me to stop. "That's Romeo. He's a bull camel. That means he's not gelded. He sires the babies. He's all male. Bulls can be very dangerous, so he has to be handled the right way. He's actually very gentle. All the females really respect him."

Romeo has muscular front legs, overdeveloped like an athlete's. "It's okay, you can get a little closer," says Gil. Romeo breaks his reverie with a sidelong glance. His dark-brown eyes are rimmed with black hair like charcoal, the impenetrable eyes of a boxer in the ring. He emanates quiet power.

"Bulls are always kept by themselves, except when the girls are in season and ready to breed," says Gil. "They're most dangerous when they're in rut and want to get at the females in heat."

I take in Romeo's strength. A bovine (cattle) bull is also a powerful beast, but squatter and lower, as I recall from my family's farm. The feeling of intimidation is similar, but this camel's train-car height makes him more awesome. A bovine bull can gore and kill you, but "a bull camel can kick and bite you to death," Gil says. Or just casually sit on you. "If they get angry at something, usually mistreatment, they just lay down on you and don't get up. You smother." A bull may suffocate another camel by lying across its neck.

"How often does he get with the females?" I ask.

"Can't say I've counted, but one bull can service a herd of twenty females."

I don't want to die at the hands, or forelegs, of a suddenly enraged camel, so I edge away. Gil shows me more camels out in the field, fondly listing their names like a father. Turns out he is. Most of the camels view him as top bull in the herd, with his wife, Nancy, as second. *Such power*, I think, to be in charge of camels.

I stop at the little farmhouse bathroom to wash my hands. There's camel milk soap by the sink, but it's curled-edge thin. I pull back the shower curtain to look for another bar. A big dark turtle shines in the bathtub, wet and unmoving in his private porcelain world.

Back in the kitchen, Nancy, a bouncy redhead, scooches her chair to the table. "So nice to meet ya!" she says. We sit down as Gil makes me chamomile tea.

Gil and Nancy explain how they met. Both are animal handlers. A graduate of the Exotic Animal Training and Management Program at Moorpark College in Southern California, Nancy trains and exhibits exotic birds. Gil came to one of her shows.

"When we met, I called him a liar," recalls Nancy, her freckled face beaming with sass. "He said he had camels, and I'd heard that before."

"Guys say that in the animal dating world?"

"They do! I'd just been out with this guy who said he had three camels. He didn't have a single one!"

"Like the 'I have a Porsche in the shop' guy?"

"I guess so! But I wasn't buying it. So I was kind of mean to Gil."

"But I told her, I really do have camels!" he says earnestly.

"And he really did!" Nancy was preparing to buy the farm, so after they had dated for two years, Gil moved his camels from Northern California to live with her — and birds and donkeys and dogs and cats. An ark of creatures inhabits their windswept place.

"You wanna see the birds?" Nancy leads me to the basement, but I stop on the old white stairs. The room reverberates with screams, squawks, and calls from a dozen birds, so loud that they hurt my ears, but Nancy's shouting cheerfully over the noise. Yellow, green, blue, and orange birds with protruding beaks and crested heads perch in airy cages or stroll across the bottoms like little kings. She moves along, describing her darlings. "Here's my beloved Kolabi the cockatoo, he's been with me forever. This is Squeak, my gorgeous, ornery Catalina macaw. First time I met Gil she chased me around the stage, laughing and biting me. This little parrot, Lola, loves to sing. She's getting ready to perform in a few weeks. And Mayan the toucan is the sweetest bird in the world!" Vivacious in her red blouse and faded blue jeans, Nancy glows, as exuberant as her feathered talkers and songstresses. They're like comrades at a vaudeville show.

"You came at a good time," she says. "Christmas is over, so the Nativity shows are done."

"What's that?"

"That's where we go out to churches or Christmas pageants with the camels and dress up. Like the manger scene from the Bible? We walk in with the camels, dressed like the Wise Men or Mary and Joseph. I'm a really good Virgin Mary!"

I can see her in a blue mantle, her smile barely repressed under a church spotlight. "And Gil goes too?"

"Usually, yeah. Sometimes we have to split up, but we'd rather not. It's nice to have a job where you can play dress-up together! And he looks good in a headdress!"

The basement counters hold a jumble of farm implements, computer parts, and paperwork. Thick brown-paper feed bags litter the floor. Shiny tools hang from a pegboard.

"Gil's working on a new camel-milk lotion right now. Like a sample?" I swipe some white cream from a little jar. It has a rustic herbal scent and no camel smell at all — not that I'd know what one would smell like. The camels actually look pretty clean, now that I think about it. No buggy eye corners, no feces encrusting the tails, no pools of liquid dung like cattle.

We go back upstairs for another mug of tea with Gil. However jovial Nancy has been, I can see that neither of them has any idea what I want, and it's too soon for them to trust me. Outwardly we are pretty different people. I live in a coastal city, haven't worked a crop since college, and the only animal I want is a horse.

I take a breath. "So I have this idea. We should think about making a dairy business somehow. I can help send you customers for camel milk. You could sell it to them. Most of their kids can't have regular milk. But they could have this. There's such a high rate of autism in California and across the country. It's increasing every year and now it's one of every 110 kids, and that's a known undercount."

I share my hope that camel milk might benefit my son and explain how I found the Israeli article. They move their chairs closer, Gil across the table, Nancy by the stove. Gil's green eyes are dark and empathetic. Nancy frowns with concentration. I finish my pitch. They don't say anything.

Gil sighs. "We've gotten calls from people about investing or trying to set up a milk business. Like I said, we pretty much decided not to meet with people about it anymore. But you're a mom and seemed sincere, so we wanted to hear more about that."

"The milk is perfectly safe, we drink it all the time. Our friends do too. But we're not sure about selling to the public," interjects Nancy. "We don't want any legal problems. What if someone's kid gets sick from something else and they sue us, God forbid? We could lose everything," she says. The land glows in the sunset through the darkening window behind her.

"I am sincere, that's for sure. Lost my career to help my son and support autism, so yeah. As far as getting sued, we could get a business insurance policy for that," I say.

"We also don't have a lot of time," says Nancy. "We'd have to stop our business and stay home, invest in a dairy. Did you see the trained turkeys outside? Right now we're on the road part of the year doing a turkey show, and bring the birds and camels, too. It's hard to get someone to watch things while we're gone."

So maybe this isn't a *farm* farm, I realize. Maybe they're more animal people than farm people.

"Do you ever want to stay home and have a dairy?"

"We think about that in the future, maybe when we're a little older or not traveling so much. But it's been this many years, and we only have two or three milking camels! It's thanks to Gil we have any! He can get camels to give milk without the babies."

"How does he do that?"

"I have a way," he says modestly, and it sounds like a trade secret, so I don't push.

Nancy gets salsa for corn chips from the fridge, revealing white bottles of lotion on shelves designed to hold ketchup. "We'd like to use camels for therapy," Gil says. "I used to do camel therapy for disabled people in Northern California. A place called Dragon Slayers. People got more confidence, better balance and strength. Camels didn't spook, so the wheelchairs didn't bother them."

"Horse riding is therapeutic for disabled kids, so why not camels?" I say.

"They have an ability to connect with humans — sometimes it's like they just know things. Like when to be calm, or slow down with people who need more time."

He pauses. "The idea of the IUD came from camels, did you know?"

"No, how?"

"An apricot pit or stone was placed in the camel's uterus so it couldn't get pregnant. That's what gave them the idea of the IUD."

Before I can ask who in the world would want camel birth control, Gil asks, "And how did you get the idea, about camel milk and autism? It's not something most people would think of. How did you find out about camel milk in the first place? Are you Jewish, or do you have some connection to camels?"

"No, nothing like that. I was talking to a camel guy at a kids' bookfair. He made soap and lotions from the milk. And he said it was nonallergenic and given in hospitals to premature babies. And I thought right then that it might help my son."

"What fair was that?"

"A fair in Orange County, near Newport Beach, where I live."

He says, "I did that fair."

And now I remember the dark-haired guy in the green hat. He'd been standing at the narrow table with the soaps. It's his camel that started my impractical mission, out here in the desert, two hours and a world away from my friends and son.

I say, "Oh, it's you."

Now I can safely tell him my miracle. "I just got some milk."

"Where from?"

"Israel."

"I'm Israeli. Wow, where did you get it? It's not really legal there."

"I know."

I tell him about my calls to Israel, about Amnon and Eyal.

"Where does Eyal live?" I name the town. Gil says his brother lives there.

They seem to like me. "Come back soon," they say. "Just call first."

"You mean people don't?"

"Sure. Lots of people try to get in and see the camels," Nancy sighs. "They come riiight up to the door and —" she pantomimes a goofy knock.

"No problem, I wasn't born in a barn," I say, smiling. Gil walks me partway out and then returns to his camels, whose regal shapes are silhouetted by the fading light.

Driving home, passing rural porch lights scattering holes in the dark, I feel energized, like I've boarded a flight to a country I've only dreamed of. I've actually *seen* camels, met people who understand them. Gil and Nancy may never sell their milk, but I will meet them and their camels again.

7 CAMEL MILK MIRACLE

"You know, I really love you guys."
— Jonah

After a year of living in our new single-parent home, Jonah is doing well some of the time. He's sweet and funny, reads, plays with toy cars, and talks about his favorite TV shows. He's made some friends at his new school for children with ADHD (attention-deficit hyper-activity disorder). But some things aren't going that great.

Every morning, after I cut up and tediously grind his meds (he can't swallow pills yet), I walk him through each daily task — brushing his teeth, washing his face, combing his hair, getting dressed. He's as slow as an old clock, distracted by an object in his room or something funny in his own head. Although he's smart and as winsome as a happy boy can be, I'm getting concerned. It's taking more effort to keep him on track these days, not less. But there's nothing else I can do.

My milk-import scheme is working. I've connected with an airport veterinarian, who clears the way at customs for a suitcase containing twenty-four bottles from Eyal. So I'm just waiting for funding for some behavioral therapy so I can get unbiased data from therapists when I give Jonah the milk. Like every therapy or need connected to autism, it's taken several meetings, and months are going by.

Around this time I meet Tony, a tall, lean, blue-eyed ex-paratrooper and former bike racer with a deeply compassionate heart. A healthcare executive, he has three teenage daughters of his own. The first time he meets Jonah, he picks us up at the airport. The second time, he comes to teach Jonah to garden and even brings him a new pair of gloves. After some cursory attention to our patio bushes, Jonah takes the shears and snips the gloves' fingers off.

"Why are you acting that way?" I hiss at him in the kitchen, but then soften and ask, "Are you nervous?"

"Is he gonna marry you and be our new stepdad?"

I'm surprised but ask, "Is that what you want?"

"Yes," he says.

"No one can be sure right now, but there's a good chance. But maybe not, if you keep acting this way! So you'd better settle down, mister." I hug him and smile.

Next time, Tony and Jonah are about to meet up in a park. "Mom, you should ask him to be your boyfriend," Jonah says, his gaze serious and his voice instructive. "If you want something in life, you have to go for it, so go over and let him know how you feel." He's very proud when Tony says yes (although he's already taken the boyfriend slot).

Tony starts quietly appearing in the mornings to help get Jonah ready for school (something I never asked him to do). He takes Jonah for walks, scans menus for dairy ingredients, and takes on the dreary pill crushing. He doesn't lose his cool when Jonah slips away from us and reappears atop a thirty-foot-high ocean wall. Tony's a tough, analytical, patient, and loving man. He hasn't been spooked by autism. He can deal with camel milk.

But something's changing with Jonah, and not for the better. He's fine at breakfast, but an hour or two later he's hyper and unreachable — unable to control himself, touching everything, kicking my seat in the car, unfocused, not there. One night at a bookstore he scales a ceiling-high ladder in seconds. Sometimes I cry in despair.

After watching our struggles, one afternoon Tony says, "Why don't you give him that milk you've been saving? What have you got to lose?"

"I need data," I begin, but I stop before the end of my sentence. Doctors aren't helping. Diet isn't helping. Therapy probably won't help much, and those hours still haven't been approved. These breakdowns are coming straight from his body, an internal mechanism he's helpless to stop.

I walk to the freezer and lay my hand on a bottle. I set it on the counter. It'll be thawed by evening.

At bedtime, Jonah's in an orange cowboy T-shirt, his hair short from a buzz cut by his dad that broke my heart. I fondle the brown bristles, soft as a shaven puppy.

I measure four ounces of camel milk into a stainless-steel cup and pour it into his cereal. "Here's your bedtime snack," I singsong, setting it on the dining room table like always.

Jonah takes his first spoonful, milk falling in drops. Then another. Tony and I sneak a quick look at each other. "You like it, honey?"

"Yes, Mom, it's good." He holds the dripping spoon high, showing off as usual.

"Look at me!" I say. He smiles, showing me his open mouth. "Not the gaping maw!" I say, our running joke as I take a photo. I lead him upstairs to the bathroom, wipe his chin, stand over him as he smears toothpaste on his brush and hops like a rabbit. He drops to the carpet to grab his stuffed dog, then reaches for his little cars.

"No, get in bed. I'll read to you." I lie next to him as he pulls his favorite book closer. "Okay, nighty night, honey."

"Night, Mom."

Downstairs, Tony has washed the bowl and spoon. He lifts the bottle and we stare at the swirling white liquid. "You're a great mother," he says, and leaves me with a hug. I collapse on the sofa and stare at the ceiling. By now I have no real expectations for the milk, just a faint hope of improvement. It's all been way too hard.

At 7 a.m. the alarm rings. I pull Jonah gently from bed, his long white legs muscular and warm, to get ready for school. "Your clothes are here," I say, pointing to the blue shirt and cargo pants, and head for the kitchen.

Tony arrives and goes to check on him. "He's doing okay. He says he'll be here in a minute."

He won't be here in a minute.

I set out Jonah's waffle and low-sugar syrup. Before the usual five-minute countdown, he's coming down the stairs. His feet aren't dragging. "Sit here, honey," I say, pointing to his chair. We adults take seats on opposite sides of the table.

Jonah picks up his knife and fork and starts cutting his waffle. I've taught him to do this many times, manipulating his fingers through the motions, but it has never really worked — until now. "Want some syrup?"

"Sure, thanks, Mom." He cuts a piece of waffle and lifts it to his mouth. His knife isn't slipping all over as usual. He's composed as he sips his watery solution of crushed-pill juice.

"You know, I really love you guys."

"You do?"

"Yes, I really do. You do so much for me. You're really great."

I sit here watching. "And Mom, you do a lot. I mean, you get me ready for school, make my food, make my medicines…"

He's looking at me, but not just at my face. Something is different. His eyes look straight into mine. They are black-lashed morning glories in the pale light.

"You're awesome," he says. He cuts a sausage link with the knife and calmly takes a bite.

I don't look at Tony. "We're glad to do it," he says. "That's really nice of you to say that you appreciate your mom."

Jonah's knife doesn't clang to the floor as usual but rests by the plate. "So what are you going to do today, Mom?" I'm dumbfounded. While he sometimes makes insightful comments or asks questions, it's not usually so easeful or about me as this.

"I guess I'll clean up the house and maybe do some paperwork."

"Who's taking me to school?"

"I will," says Tony, staring at him.

"And who's picking me up?"

"Uhh, I will," I say.

Jonah eats without jamming big pieces into his mouth or splattering the table with syrup. There's no rolling his head on his collar or saying things to himself.

"It's time to go to school," he says. "We don't want to be late."
He gets off the chair, and instead of smashing his feet into his shoes
as usual, he attaches the fasteners and puts his own backpack on. He
stands by the table like a little prince, waiting expectantly.

"Love you," I say, and pull his head to my chest.

"Love you too, Mom." Tony grabs his keys, and they're gone. I
stand in the entry hall. What have I seen?

Tony returns to the condo.

"How was he on the way to school?" He's been known to grab
door handles, press his feet on the dashboard.

"He was fine. He got out and didn't forget his backpack."

We look at each other. "So did you notice anything?" I say.

"He was totally different!"

"Like how?"

"Well for one, he was talking to me for the first time! Like he just
realized I'm an actual person. Not just gabbing about whatever comes
in his head."

"Okay. Did he look at your eyes?"

"Yeah, he did! It was kind of — great. He hasn't looked right at me
before," Tony says.

"And how about what he said?"

"I've never heard him say anything like that. I wasn't sure he was
capable of it. I'm amazed. What about you?"

I hesitate. What just happened seems so incredible that I want to be
careful about it, like handling a painted egg or describing light from a
cathedral window.

"He was so much better. He came down dressed. He walked better
too. When he said how much he loved us, and what we did for him, I
couldn't believe it. I know he loves me, he's said it, but never like today.
So emotional! And he looked right at me. That's hard, but he did it
naturally," I say.

"We didn't even ask him anything. He just talked! And in actual
paragraphs too, not cartoon talk. And he didn't get food all over the
table. That alone is a miracle," Tony says.

"He also said it was time to go to school. And didn't half-slide off his chair like usual. And got his own shoes! I always have to remind him about shoes."

"And the backpack. Usually I get the backpack," adds Tony. "How much did you give him?"

"Four ounces."

"Better give it to him again tonight!"

"I will."

Tony shakes his head.

As the hours pass, I wonder how school's going. I can't really call over and say I gave him camel milk and want to know if it's working. Plus the few people I've told of my camel milk idea always think I'm saying "chamomile" like the tea. Anyway, it's got to be our secret, so teachers can give me feedback without bias. Without the therapists, that's as scientific as I can get.

After school, Jonah climbs into the car more quickly, less slow-limbed than usual. His backpack is on, not lugged behind him by a teacher's aide. On the ride he answers a few questions and keeps his feet to himself. At home, he sits nicely for a snack. Tony arrives. "Hey, how ya doing?" he says to my son.

"Hi. Okay," he replies. At dinner he eats neatly and sits upright. He looks briefly into my eyes a couple of times. We talk about school. "It was okay."

"Did you have any trouble?"

"No," he says. "Kaira got in trouble and had to go to the quiet room."

At bedtime, I take the bottle of milk from the fridge with awe. I pour four ounces, just like before.

I realize there's been another change. In the past, cow milk made Jonah very restless, like other dairy-intolerant autistic kids I've known. "He slept all night last night," I whisper to Tony.

Upstairs my boy goes, without dragging his feet or playing on the handrails. In bed, he calls, "Night, Mom."

On day 3, we walk through a parking lot with my hand on Jonah's jacket collar, but he pulls away and keeps walking. Instead of veering in front of me, he actually stays with us. At a light, I hold his sleeve.

"Let go, Mom," he says. The sign flashes "Walk," and he steps out first, turning his head awkwardly to check for cars.

Back home, we take off our jackets. "Want to watch TV?"

"Sure, okay." When the cartoons come on, he bounces on the sofa but doesn't jump on it.

"This is really shocking," says Tony.

"I know! I hoped I'd see something, but I never expected *this*."

He says, "It's like he's fully formed now."

Every day we pour the milk. Every day Jonah is better.

There are technical terms to sum up the first days of Jonah's drinking camel milk: fine-motor improvements (cutting, eating, tying shoes); better executive functioning (remembering to get his backpack, asking about the school and pickup schedule); enhanced motor planning (better walking and climbing, awareness of streets, staying with the group, watching for cars); increased attention (focus on people and environment); greater empathy ("You do so much for me, you're really great"); a slight increase in eye contact; an increase in emotional speech ("I really love you guys, you're awesome"); improved theory of mind (thinking about other people's thoughts and how they view things differently than he does). But overall the effect is more than that. He's more fluid, social, and attuned.

It's amazing to see him doing so much better. Nothing is this easy in autism.

And the best part is seeing more of who he is.

Hail to a bottle of milk.

8 THE MILK KNOWS NO BORDERS

"He's a different kid."
— TONY

Amnon is quietly astonished by the results I report to him. This could be a scientifically important insight, he says. Together we expand on our initial hypothesis that camel milk can reduce inflammation, and that immune system dysfunction is present in some cases of autism. "So if he's doing this well on four ounces, let's take it to eight," he says. "The same amount as the Crohn's disease patients."

I'm hoping, like Amnon, that a larger amount might lead to even more improvement. Can it do that? How much is too much?

That night I fill a cup with eight ounces of camel milk, and Jonah drinks it down. The next two days, same story. He's bright-eyed and looking good. But as he's doing homework after school, his right arm jerks. Then again. He seems unaware of it. "Are you doing your work?" I ask.

"Yes, Mom."

The next day, the same arm jerks again, forming an L shape as it wings from his body. Then his mouth twists open, as if he's feeling an itch or a sting. I've never seen this before.

"Do you have a cold or an itch?"

"No, I'm not sick," he says.

Soon he grimaces again, like he wants to let something out.

"Darn it, what is that? His arm is jerking, and now he's making these weird grimaces," I tell Tony. "Do you see that?"

It's impossible not to. The arm contortions happen every other hour, the grimaces a few times a day. Otherwise he's the same.

Amnon has never heard of this. "That's a unusual reaction."

"My son's all about unusual," I remind him.

After two more days, I cut Jonah's serving back to four ounces. The jerks and grimaces stop.

One morning I stare at a half-full bottle when I'm alone. The white paste forms little snowdrifts under the rim. That's supposed to be full of good things, says Eyal. But right now I'll just try the liquid milk. I pour two ounces into a little cup and drink it fast. It tastes like thick nothing. A wave of sensation spreads across my brain. *Whoosh.* I wonder if I should grab the fridge handle to steady myself, but my vision and balance are fine. It's painless, not euphoric. After a full minute, it recedes and is gone.

This milk must be powerful.

My friendly vet at Los Angeles Airport is getting nervous. "I think you should call the higher-ups. Make sure they're okay with it."

This scares me. "I'll think about it," I say. He's been so nice. But if his superiors say no to my bringing it in, I'm screwed.

I've researched the commercial permit process for importing milk, a mess of codes describing all manner of fish, fowl, feathers, and meat. During my career I've waded through aerospace specifications, defense appropriations, state law, disability law, and medical literature, but this stuff is virtually unreadable. It's sections of jargon, lists of gruesome animal and bug parts. Most people who deal with this are professionals, but I don't have the money to hire an expert. The milk is already costing me seven hundred dollars a load. So I ignore the vet's hints.

After two months of drinking the milk, Jonah's cheeks are smooth. The white bumps are gone, along with the chicken-bump skin on the back of his arms. The behavior breakdowns stopped when he started the milk. He still needs some reminding to complete tasks, but he no longer plummets to the behavioral abyss. The new school's reports are good, and he's tested with a college-level vocabulary. The camel milk has expanded his language, added emotional content, and made our chats less one-sided.

I drag out his therapy binders and view previous skill tests. I assign percentages to his progress. When I'm done, I estimate that his autism symptoms have diminished by 30 percent.

Tony says, "I haven't known him as long as you, but that sounds right. The change is clear. He's a different kid."

"I think he's the same kid, just one that can control himself better. Even his motor skills have improved. I never expected that."

"He's not losing it anymore like he was," he says.

"And he's getting calcium from real animal milk, not just potato milk. I hope it gives his bones a good foundation. And his skin shows the milk is acting systemically, fixing something inside."

"How long do we have to keep giving it to him?"

"I don't know. No one knows. He's a test case!" I laugh. I'm happy, in love with camel milk. It's so great to pour the milk into his cup, knowing how much it's helping. Flying those heavy bottles into the country like gold bars is worth it. This is some kind of miracle.

Finally, I learn of a teeny exception to the laws barring noncommercial importation of milk. You can bring in milk for a child's personal use. The exception is probably not intended for long-term use. But I'll argue that interpretation should be in the best interests of the child, if anyone asks. In the meantime, I'll keep bringing it in.

But the next time I call the vet at LAX, he says, "You really need to call."

"Who would I call? Can you give me a name of someone friendly, that you know will approve it?"

"Just call the USDA in Washington."

"Don't you have any contacts there?"

"Nah, that's a whole different ball game."

The Israeli family with whom I initially shared the shipments has had great success with camel milk. As soon as they gave it to their four-year-old boy, his frequent bowel bleeding stopped. But now they're only bringing in enough milk for him (though we still lend bottles to each other in an emergency), so I'm on my own. And I'm planning a big order: forty-eight frozen bottles, heavy as a church bell, my biggest buy yet.

And now I need a courier. Amnon's daughter Tal volunteers to do it if I buy the ticket, which will cost $1,400.

So I take a deep breath and call the USDA in Washington. The soft-voiced woman I'm transferred to tells me I'll need two letters, one describing the situation and one from Jonah's doctor.

"Okay."

"There are no guarantees it'll be approved," she cautions. "The decision will have to be made by other people."

The last time we visited Jonah's longtime autism doctor, he was very pleased with his blood work and performance. So I told him about the milk.

"Chamomile?"

"No, camel milk. Milk from a camel. It made him function so much better," I whispered, always careful not to talk too much about my son's issues in front of him. Jonah was standing slightly away from us.

"I don't believe it," the doctor said.

"Why not? People have been using it for thousands of years for health issues."

"Because I never heard of it."

"It's not very known in this country. And it is helping — our visit today shows it."

"I've been practicing for twenty-five years, and if I haven't heard of it, it doesn't work."

"But no one can know everything. It doesn't mean something is useless if you don't know about it."

"Yes, it does."

Then he leaned forward, his eyes hot, and said, "If you think camel milk helps autism, you're stupid."

"Doctor, you called my mom stupid!" said Jonah, his eyes wide. "You can't call her stupid! That's bad. You need to say you're sorry."

"Well, it's just...it's not possible — your mom..."

I looked at him, his choleric face pink from vexation. I'd hoped a brilliant outside-the-box thinker like him would be interested. And then it hit me: *We don't need him anymore.*

I call another of Jonah's doctors. She's an MD with an integrative practice, blending traditional medicine with diet advice and carefully chosen supplements. She'll write the letter.

I send it off to the USDA, and within days I get a call from the 202 area code. "We've made a decision," says the woman I talked to before. The milk will be allowed through. "We authorized twenty-four bottles."

Oh, I'm so happy. But I need a double quantity. "I hate to ask. But I have to pay for the full airline ticket whether I'm bringing in one suitcase or more. Can I get two?"

That requires another decision. Days pass. I check back.

Forty-eight bottles will be on their way.

9 CAMELS

A God-Given Marvel?

"Will they not look at the camels, how they are created?"
— Qur'an 88:17

I've learned a lot about camels now. And they are some crazy animals. They look comical, even slow, with long legs and floppy feet. Their sex-kitten eyelashes and kooky humps appear drawn by a caricaturist's hand. Their heads swivel in all directions atop their long, thick necks. They extrude grassy little poops like hamster droppings. With soft hair and naturally "smiley" faces, they could be stuffed animals come to life.

But the fun is just a disguise. This majestic beast is a Darwinist champion, a testament to the survival of the fittest. Behind the funny image is an animal perfect for its harsh environment.

Everyone knows camels can go for weeks without water — in fact, it's the only thing most people know about them. But the humps are not water tanks (they contain up to eighty pounds of fat), so how do they do it? They sweat very little, even in desert temperatures of 120°F or more, because their sweat glands are deeper and more scattered than those of other animals. Grooves in their nostrils funnel moisture from their breath back to their mouths. Their thick coats and tough skin offer insulation from the heat. As they safely dehydrate in challenging conditions, they can lose up to 40 percent of their body weight in water. Oval blood cells (camelids are the only mammals to have them) keep their blood circulating through constricted blood vessels and carry vital oxygen. These cells can rehydrate to 240 percent of their original volume, significantly more than other animals' typical 150 percent, letting camels quickly recover from water deprivation. Such extreme rehydration can burst the blood cells of other animals.

Viewed piece by piece, camels look like a bad puzzle. But they have the last laugh. Those long legs keep their bodies raised above scorchingly hot desert sand. Their wide, padded feet (don't look up "camel toes" on the internet unless you want to see the human version) keep them stable on shifting sands and rocks. In a sandstorm, their nostrils close, and a third, clear eyelid protects their eyes from blowing sand. Their velvet lips, the upper lip naturally split, can munch tough thorns and plants. A goat's got nothing on them.

For baby camels and hungry nomads, the best adaptation may be the way females let down their milk. They can reportedly deliver their stored milk in ninety seconds, for efficient nursing in bad conditions. Come wind, come rain, the kitchen's open.

Although camels can go for a month without water, they can still die from thirst. Keeping them watered is an important duty in herding families. Thirsty camels can drink up to thirty gallons of water in thirteen minutes.

There are two kinds of camels: the smooth-haired, one-humped dromedary of the Arab world, a desert dweller; and the shaggy two-humped Bactrian, living mainly on the Asian steppes and in mountains. Dromedaries greatly outnumber Bactrians. I remember the difference this way: the Bactrian's double humps resemble the letter B, and a dromedary's single hump looks like a D. Camels are part of the Camelidae family, which includes wild and domestic Bactrians, dromedaries, llamas, guanacos, alpacas, and vicunas. Unlike other ruminants such as cattle and sheep, camelids have three distinct stomach compartments instead of four. They eat foliage off trees, not just the ground, chewing their food and regurgitating it in a cud. Even though they're herbivorous, camels have been known to eat fish — an unpleasant sight for the bystander when a cud regurgitates like a fishy plug of tobacco.

Camels can weigh up to 1,600 pounds and stand more than seven feet tall. They hang out in flocks or caravans, although Gil calls his camels a herd. Except for a few endangered flocks of wild Chinese-Mongolian Bactrians, most camels today are domesticated. (Australia's feral camels annoy farmers by eating and trampling things.) Unlike horses, camels walk by moving both legs on the same side at the same time, in a gait called a pace. This makes them rock and sway under riders, one reason for their nickname "ship of the desert." Even so, their energy requirements for walking and load bearing are lower than scientists expect; such efficiency lets these creatures survive in their hot homelands.

The camel is the rare livestock animal that's also prestigious. Camels have been traded, branded, raced, ridden, adorned, artificially inseminated, roasted, milked, and even cloned. Although they surprisingly originated in North America around forty-five million years ago (some fossils have been found on Los Angeles's glamorous Wilshire Boulevard), they're Eastern, Asian, and African cultural icons. From the popular camel-racing tracks of the United Arab Emirates to the colorful Pushkar Camel Fair in India, from the roadside camel milk stands of Chad to the pyramid tourist rides in Egypt, camels meet human needs that other animals can't. They've served as trucks, companions, pharmacies, and portable pantries for ages, especially for nomadic peoples, or pastoralists.

Amnon says the Tarabin Bedouins (or al-Tirabin) supply Eyal with camels. This nomadic population of about half a million lives in the Negev Desert near Eyal, and through the Sinai Peninsula, Egypt, and beyond. The Negev faction of around 160,000 people claims descent from the tribe of the Prophet Mohammed.

Once this mighty land of crags, craters, dunes, and streams belonged only to those who could endure its rugged beauty. Through it, merchants transported spices and other goods on camels, covering thirty-five kilometers (about twenty-two miles) a day, a typical range for a camel, on their way to Mediterranean ports. The local Tarabin herded camels, sheep, and goats over plains and wadis (gullies that fill with water when it rains). They have a reputation as outstanding hosts and fierce fighters. Tarabin men kept — and often still keep — women at home, without schooling, to tend hearth and flock.

After centuries of ranging freely on this land, these people now can't prove legal ownership of it. Israel has tried to "sedentarize" many Bedouin over the years, stopping their flocks from grazing and pushing their owners into living in towns (thus preserving the Negev for its new owners). But apparently it's hard to kill the nomadic spirit. Over half the Negev's Tarabin still live in unrecognized settlements, though perhaps not in goatskin tents, and their birth rate is high (over seven kids per woman). Since their allegiance is mostly to the tribe, not the state, their cultural assets like camels remain off the grid, thwarted by rules and limits. I do not know anything about Bedouins, Middle East politics, or tribal resistance, but I think these herders and their animals should survive.

At least the Muslims I've been meeting know camels aren't that strange. "Camel milk is in the Holy Qur'an," they say excitedly. Although camels were domesticated long before the rise of Islam, they're enshrined in a hadith, an account of the Prophet's experience that provides guidance for Islamic life. And it's not just the milk that's divine. The website Islam Question and Answer includes this advice:

> Q. I hope that you can provide me with a scientific answer — if such knowledge is available — about the saheeh hadeeth about drinking camel's urine. May Allaah reward you.
>
> A. Praise be to Allaah. The hadeeth...says that some people came to Madeenah and fell sick. The Prophet (peace and blessings of Allaah be upon him) told them to drink the milk and urine of camels, and they recovered and grew fat.... The health benefits of drinking the milk and urine of camels...are many, [are] known to the earlier generations of medical science and...have been proven by modern scientific research.

Some might scoff at the idea of superpowered camel pee, but since pharmaceutical companies use mare's urine to make the drug Premarin for menopausal women, we know that urine may have some therapeutic properties.

The Qur'an details the great camel gift explicitly. "Will they not look at the camels, how they are created?" (88:17). "As for the camels, We have made them of the signs of the religion of Allah for you... when they fall down eat of them, and feed the poor man who is contented and the beggar; thus have We made them subservient to you, that you may be grateful" (22:36).

The Qur'an dictates that camels are to be respected and their gifts shared with the sick (like my son, I reflect) and the hungry. An oral Arab and nomadic Muslim proverb says Allah shared ninety-nine of his names with humanity, but only the camel knows the hundredth name. Other versions say the camel smiles because he knows the ninety-nine names, or because he knows the secret one. Ask a different group, you get a different answer, including the claim that it's not true at all.

What I know is this: while camels seem funny, elegant, and intimidating, I feel deep reverence when their milk is in my hands.

10 FORTY-EIGHT BOTTLES OF MILK IN THE FRIDGE

"Are they all...gone?"

— ME TO TONY

I drive to LAX and collect my two giant suitcases of milk. I've bought an upright freezer for my garage to give the bottles their own special home.

Not long after, Tony, who's now my fiancé, takes me to visit England, his home country, while Jonah is staying with his father. So I take a break from camels and their milk and lift my eyes to the world. In London, I try a Scotch egg, biting through the crumb-covered sausage to the cooked yolk inside. Plump, pale blue-eyed people who resemble my relatives stroll through a grassy park. But the reach of desert culture extends even here. The famed Harrods department store is dotted with women in black *abayas* trimmed with Swarovski crystals, their exclusive handbags, watches, and sunglasses more visible than their faces.

When we arrive back home after the trip, I flick the garage light switch. It doesn't come on. "What happened, did my light bulb burn out?"

He checks the bulb, and it's fine. "I'll look at the breakers," he says. The condo's inside electrical breaker panel is okay. So we go in the garage and spy a breaker panel I didn't know I had, with one flipped switch. It's warm in here. I go over to the freezer that holds the big new load of camel milk I stored before our trip, open the door, and scream.

45

Tony comes running. I turn away, holding my forehead, covering my eyes. He looks in the freezer and says, "Aw, damn it."

"Are they all…gone?" I ask.

He looks in the freezer again. "Sweetheart, just go inside. Let me deal with this."

I stand stock-still, afraid to look again.

"I think I can save a few," he calls, hope in his voice. But inside I just know there is none.

I saw green mold crawling over the bottles. I saw milk yellowed to a putrid hue of decay. I saw things no camel milk lover should ever see. I saw two thousand dollars wasted. My heart tumbles to the floor with grief. "Can we even save the freezer?" I say miserably.

"I think so," Tony says. One by one he chucks the stinking milk bottles into a plastic trash can, their dull thud echoing against the side. Leaning my head on the doorframe, I think of the countdown song I sang with other kids on school buses to pass the time. "Ninety-nine bottles of beer on the wall, ninety-nine bottles of beer, take one down, pass it around, ninety-eight bottles of beer on the wall…" With each thump, the tune plays mournfully in my head. "Forty-eight bottles of milk on the shelf, going, going away."

Tony gives the freezer a scrub, I give it another. But no quantity of baking soda will banish the foul smell embedded in its plastic lining.

So what now? I call Gil and confess what happened. He and Nancy are going to Israel, and he offers to bring milk back if I pay half his airfare. For me it's a steal. I introduce him to Eyal, who coincidentally lives not only in the same town as Gil's brother, but right next door. Gil takes the doctor's letter explaining my son's need for milk. From Israel to America, every official waves him through, sending their blessings to mother and child.

The Tarabin Bedouins have replenished my stock of milk. The *on* indicator of the new freezer glows red in the rewired garage. Forty-eight bottles of milk in the fridge, many acts of care.

There's goodness flowing through this milk.

11 GETTING CLOSE TO CAMELS

"The camels know who to listen to."

— GIL RIEGLER

Big blond Camelot stands peacefully with his nose under mine on a windy day at Oasis Camel Dairy. I've come to pick up some milk and spend time with the camels. Today the ranch is a green-brown dreamscape with an improbable smear of camel in the foreground. The herd mills slowly in the pasture: camels retain an air of stillness even when moving quickly. As the biggest, strongest camel on the lot, Camelot is the obvious candidate for herd leader, but he's the lowest of the low. Even baby camels run after him, taunting him like an overgrown schoolboy. Today he looks downright hangdog, with ragged patches of hair peeling like a beloved stuffed animal (he's molting). "He doesn't know he's big and strong," says Gil, petting him.

If not Camelot, who is the boss dromedary? Today, it's pregnant Belina, but even three other females outrank him. Still, he may yet have a chance. "It always changes, who decides to be bossy that day. But the camels know who to listen to," Gil says.

Just then, Camelot puts his nose close to a white camel's face. She shows her teeth, a quick gesture of aggression, and his head veers back. She regards him with black-rimmed doll eyes, her smile unchanged. "She just told him to knock it off, and he did," says Gil. Languidly she turns away, and a chastened Camelot eventually leaves too, his lower lip straight, not hanging in the pout that shows a camel's contentment.

Out here in Ramona, the turkey flock, which chases red, grain-filled trucks in shows at county fairs, choreographs its movements with mass gobbles that fill the air. Their high-pitched chuckles punctuate the groans and sighs of the camels. I'm trying to overcome my nervousness around the camels. They're so big. Their necks curve like tree trunks or tractor tires. Their eyes don't reveal their thoughts, to me at least. And their sides bulge like boulders. If they step on my foot, like I've had ponies do, I hope their feet feel softer than a horse's.

Gil is relaxed. With his tan cheeks, arched nose, curved lips, and wide, gentle eyes, he shares some traits with his camels. Though some tower two feet above his head, he's obviously among loved ones, and not at all scared. I want to know how this works.

"So camels always have a social structure?"

"Absolutely. A well-bred camel needs either a herd or parent figure to show it who's boss, don't let it be an idiot," Gil explains affectionately. "Bottle-fed babies are the ones we worry about. You have to discipline them just like the herd would." When animals are sold young, after weaning, they're called bottle babies. Breeders both love and decry the practice. Without a herd to socialize the babies, the buyers must fulfill the role of disciplinarian. Those who can't will get run over by their camels, much as overly indulgent parents can produce spoiled teenagers.

But dominance is fluid within a herd. One camel will drape its neck over another's to show superiority. Or one camel will stand over a lying camel, straddling it with splayed feet, their heads facing the same direction like entangled twins in utero. "But they're not evil to each other. They communicate quickly and efficiently," Gil says. A fast nip to the nose is an instant correction. A newcomer may be neglected if it doesn't blend in.

A pregnant camel may reveal her condition early by distancing herself from all the dominance shenanigans. I've seen one out in the field, tail up in a "flag" position (another pregnancy sign), her back to the rocks, facing down a herd of playful adolescent males. Her face said, "I've got this, but if you touch me you're dead."

There's a strong matriarchal streak in camel social dynamics. Despite the raging strength of the bulls, daily power lies more with the females. "A young bull can shove everyone where he wants them to go. A dominant bull can move the herd, and no one gives him problems," says Gil, but "there's usually a female who takes charge, moving them around." And the older, smaller, scrappy females often assume command. Females with stronger hormones or those in season might get more assertive. But the reason Gil can get the milk without the babies, I learn, is because they attach so strongly to him.

I reach out and pat a huge camel. I hold my palm flat and offer him some grain. He takes it like a favor, with hovering, whiskered lips. I press my hand to his neck. It feels warm, smooth, and slightly stiff, like pony-hair shoes.

"Go ahead," says Gil, gesturing to the pasture. The camels out here are not that interested in me, as I don't have a grain bucket, but Gil does. "Cush, cush," says Gil, and a camel drops knobbly-kneed to the ground, front end first. Its rear end follows, folding down like an ironing board. It lies serenely, front legs tucked under its chest. "Go ahead, you can touch him."

I touch him, then stroke his back. I'm tolerated. I kneel in the poop-pebbled dirt and fondle his mane. He feels like a big sofa. I want to lean against his side, curl under his vast rib cage, and nap. I put my arm on his body and feel his warm, hairy hump through my sleeve. Then suddenly his head is in my face, and I leap up in alarm. "It's okay," says Gil, in the same voice he uses with the camels. "He's fine. You can sit next to him."

I take a breath and crouch again. His hair, like mine, is the gold of late-summer leaves, and my sunglasses match the amber of his eyes. The other camels aren't far off, and I keep looking to see if they're going to do something camelish, like bite me. Two camels walk closer, do the equivalent of a dog sniff, and zigzag away. I stroke my new friend, fingering the coarse strands springing from his dust-powdered mane. I feel like we should talk.

My mind says, "I'm honored to know you, your females' milk is more precious than rubies, I want to bring your gifts to everyone" or something like that. But all I can manage is, "Hey, guy, how are you? You're a good guy."

As I stand, the others edge over, heads sideways, as if listening to a weather report. They don't appear to see me, but their ears seem to be turned in my direction. They have a curiously immobile quality, like statuary. I walk toward the group, and one arcs away. The others wait, then make up their minds and trot off. I can barely sense the thud of their padded leathery feet. They leave no prints, like horses do. The comparison with horses crumbles further with every moment I spend with them. Horses sometimes share space with the camels here, but the animals recognize the difference and form separate herds.

Gil and I walk toward the barn. He's smiling, fully at home here as camel caretaker, getting as much as he gives in a way I don't understand.

"Gil, why do you do this?"

He sets the grain bucket over the fence. "It's just what I am supposed to do."

"How did you find out about them?"

His eyes grow darker and soften with memory. "I'd never been around camels. I'd only seen them in zoos, until I had a compulsion to be around them."

"How did that happen?"

"I was in the Israeli army," he says. "I wanted to work with animals, so when I became a commander, I found out about a base that had camels, near the Egyptian border in the south." In 1982, his unit was assigned to catch arms smugglers coming through the desert of the Sinai Peninsula, bound for Israel. "When we found camel tracks, we'd start tracking them with a Bedouin camel handler. He could look at the ground, just the faintest, almost invisible things, and say, you are tracking six camels, they have a load of this size, with this many people. He helped us find them. Sometimes we'd get a helicopter and find them in the mountains, but mostly they'd park in a Bedouin settlement and we'd confiscate their weapons and the camels.

"One night, we found seven camels. The other guys were busy, and it was up to me to get them to base. I had never in my life led a camel, done anything with them. I didn't even have a rope! I just looked at them and spoke to them. The first one followed me, and the rest came along. We walked all the way that night. When we got there, I turned on the water and everybody drank, and then they walked back with me to settle for the night. It was lucky, because I didn't know what else to do!"

The work was a natural fit for Gil. Soon he began leading groups of twenty to thirty camels for hours across the desert, riding one with the others following in a line. After leaving the army, he moved back to Canada, where he'd been born. But the cold drove him to hitchhike to the United States. "I was twenty-three, with $150 in my pocket, a guitar and a backpack. It was a spiritual journey. I told myself, wherever I end up is the right place for me."

Arriving in California, he had a feeling this was his destination. "I called my only contact, and they had a job for me. I showed up at this nice place and noticed the secretary was naked. The manager had his shirt off. I had no idea it was a clothing-optional place, but they'd just fired a person that morning. I did gardening, maintenance — it was a beautiful family location. Then I made granola and candy at a factory. Later I learned to cut very precise crystals for a brilliant engineer named Dr. Marcel Vogel. That's how I saved money to buy camels. First I bought four babies for ten thousand dollars. Then for another ten thousand, I got two females and one bull. I still do it. Vogel-cut crystals are in high demand." He points to a little trailer near the field, his cutting shed for the crystals that some people believe have special energy.

Gil paired his crystal cutting with volunteer work at Dragon Slayers, a therapy facility for physically handicapped people in Santa Cruz. "I learned to train animals, from birds to camels, horses, donkeys, mules, parrots. Even ravens and tortoises. The students learn to ride horses, drive pony carts, and do shows. It improves their balance and strength. Here they are, working with a beautiful animal, and people are interested in what they have to say."

"So why camels instead of horses, or birds?"

"The owner got a female camel named Sahara. I walked up to her in her pen, and we looked into each other's eyes. A little voice came into my head and said, as long as you have camels in your life, it will be a good one."

He pauses. "Up until then I was just searching, always wondering, what am I going to do with my life, what am I going to do? It was a switch. It just clicked."

It was an instant success. Gil credits his mentor's gentle way of training. "The animal always lets you know the next step. It's a very quiet, respectful interaction. I carry it into my own training."

The wind cuts cold over the yard as the sun suddenly drops. The turkeys gobble "chucka-chucka-chucka" in unison. I know Gil should send me packing, as there are animals to feed, soap to cut, a lotion to test, a costume to make. And it's time for me to go home. But somehow I'm reluctant to leave. He's not just a farmer, he's an animal mystic. And he's willing to share his herd with me, another creature who showed up unexpectedly.

12 HEALING WITH CAMEL MILK

"I'm so sorry, but that was amazing!"
— A FRIEND

Sometimes the phone rings and it's a woman I've never met. She's always a mother — from Israel, from Canada, from Beverly Hills. She's heard about me from Eyal or Amnon, and she's desperate. Is it true that camel milk helped your child? How much do you give him? What should I do?

What should I do, what should I do? The universal cry of the sick child's mom. Abandoned by hasty medical personnel who avoid mysterious diseases and conditions, she breaks treatment ground herself. I bear witness to her trauma, tell her what I did, add some tips. Then she gets the milk from Eyal or someone else and disappears into the ether. Eyal or Amnon usually tell me that it helped, but there's no easy way for me to keep in touch.

While the rate of autism is rising sharply, I don't know anyone else who uses camel milk. I *want* people to use it. I tell all my friends, because it's such an easy thing to do for such life-changing results. Some of them opt for expensive, out-there therapies that are far more invasive and take months. Right now I don't want to write about camel milk, though — I'm afraid that if too many people hear about it, some will be reckless about importing and get it banned by customs. That could risk Jonah's supply. And without it I'd be desperate. Now that he's back at a regular school, he especially needs to stay on an even keel.

Every time he eats too much bread, or the cookies, fruit, and pizza always offered to schoolkids, he gets wild — wacky and uncontrollable. Around fall holidays, when candy is abundant and the California air is dry, the skin around his lips breaks out in a "yeast rash" triggered by sugar. But after four ounces of camel milk, he's back to normal in no time.

Tony and I rent a house where all four kids live with us. We get married and take a honeymoon to Dubai and India. I learn at the airport that Jonah will be staying full-time with his dad, which disrupts the care plan I'd made. I'd left camel milk for Jonah, but he won't get it now. Before we head home, I get a phone call from his father. He says Jonah's behavior has deteriorated and he could lose his mainstream classroom placement and be moved to special ed. I call the teacher, who kindly says we'll address it when I get back. On my return, I gasp at the crusty sores around his beautiful pink lips. Jonah's so ashamed that he covers them with black electrical tape for Halloween trick-or-treating, but when he glimpses his reflection in a mirror, he cries and refuses to go. It's devastating. But I give him four ounces of raw camel milk, and his behavior improves right away. The sores heal in four days, without leaving the scars I'd feared.

Time passes, and we're able to buy our own house. Now Jonah's in middle school. One night one of my stepdaughter's friends comes over with a box of nickel-size crackers. "Want some?" she asks us.

"Do they have dairy?"

She reads the box. "No, they don't." Jonah eats seven as we watch television. An hour later, he goes to bed.

An hour later, he comes downstairs. "I can't sleep," he says. "My stomach hurts."

I look suspiciously at the box. In tiny print the label says "nonfat milk powder." He groans, bent over in the dining room chair, blanket draped around him. I give him half a cup of camel milk and in fifteen minutes, the pain is gone. Back upstairs he goes. The friend is astonished. "I'm so sorry," she says. "But that was amazing!"

Another time Jonah goes to a movie with other boys. He comes home and starts laughing wildly at the dinner table, then gets very belligerent and oppositional.

"Go get ready for bed now, honey." He ignores me, giddy as a drunken frat boy.

"Get up."

He looks at me, glazed and defiant.

"What did you eat at the movies?" I always send his dairy-free popcorn along.

"I ate the popcorn," he says.

"What else?" I interrogate him like a crime detective.

"I had a drink."

"How big?"

"A extra-large diet cola."

He'd never reacted to a small amount of this drink, but he'd never had this much. *Can camel milk work for this?* I wonder. It's diet, not real sugar. I fetch him four ounces of milk. After ten minutes, he's still rowdy. After thirteen, he seems calmer. After fifteen, he starts crying. "Mom, I'm sorry. I don't know why I acted like that! I feel better now. I didn't mean it." Tears run down his cheeks. He's completely calm now, like a drunk waking up sober.

So to protect my supply of camel milk, like a drug addict or an alcoholic, I keep the secret from the general public. I offer the milk to close friends, but they're nervous. One tries it on her autistic son, and his pale face briefly turns bright red. That could mean that it's working, or that he's reacting to the milk or an allergen it contains, but it scares her. Some people ask enough questions to get me to talk. Some scoff, some are astonished, some just don't believe that it works. At a party, I see a married couple roll their eyes. But ridicule means nothing to me.

Ever since I realized something wasn't right with Jonah, people, especially men, have told me I'm wrong. Or they've dismissed my efforts: "If you think that diet helps, whatever." If I'd listened to these people, his amazing progress wouldn't have happened. This attitude is part of a widespread disregard for women's opinions, which gets worse when you enter motherhood. Add the label of "special-needs mom," and people place you at preschool level. Camel milk sounds silly to these types, but autism has made me impervious, and I don't care what they think.

I meet more camel people. Riding a camel at a Renaissance Fair, I befriend another Tuareg selling silver jewelry, who knows Elhadji, my first Tuareg acquaintance from the house party. (Tip: If you meet a tall Tuareg man in robes selling silver jewelry, he might know the other Tuareg men in robes selling jewelry.) We talk on the phone about the camel salt caravans and other wonders of his world, like how his friend saw a herd of five thousand camels for sale, the size of a lake. I read old books, monitor research on PubMed, study science. I gather observations from the few kids drinking camel milk (they're all good). I half-write a business plan to start a camel dairy that would require two million dollars (an obvious pipe dream). I call the USDA to discuss importing camels (imports are unofficially barred from all but five countries to keep out diseases, although camels don't even get some of the sicknesses the agency lists as threats). I help special-needs families get therapy and school services. Life is full with Jonah's school and homework, singing, sewing, and art lessons, as I teach him to shoot a basketball, throw a football, and do chores.

The days roll on, full and filled with love. I co-parent Tony's pretty teenage girls as we blend our family. They take him to the beach and help babysit when we travel. They're mostly patient with Jonah, quashing his boyishness with sisterly rough-and-tumble. They make him wait for his turn to talk, something he learns pretty quickly. We share holidays, dinners, school projects, and graduations. I have a great husband, and everyone has more love.

In this manner, two years pass.

When Facebook becomes popular, I sign up, but my camel connections are made in real life — until I stumble across a tiny new Facebook group called Healing with Camel Milk. They're talking about using Amish camel milk. This is a revelation.

When I join the group, a man named Troyer makes mean, ungrammatical remarks in response to my first short post. I don't know this person. I write to the group's owners, explaining why I'm interested in the milk, and one, Jessica, seems wary and cool. Eventually I figure out why. Marlin Troyer is an actual Amish camel farmer. Paranoid on behalf of the group, he'd told her I was a spy for an eccentric lady he doesn't get along with, who dresses in robes and loves camels. Who are these crazy people?

Troyer finally accepts that I'm not a plant, but he's still self-righteous and unfriendly to me in his posts. Jessica, on the other hand, is now very nice. She heard about camel milk about six years after I did. One of her sons was diagnosed with autism. The other had severe eczema, speech delay, and dairy intolerance. Both were underweight and labeled as "failing to thrive." She didn't know about camel milk's healing properties; she simply wanted raw milk, which she had heard was antibacterial and antiviral. A local Amish farmer had just started milking camels, so she sent her husband to get some.

Like Jonah, her boys improved rapidly. Both drank a pint per day, and the most underweight child gained three pounds in three days; his speech also improved dramatically. After twenty-four days, the child with autism lost his tics, anger, tantrums, aggression, itching, and poor sleep, she said. So she started the Facebook group with her friend Nicole.

If this American milk works for Jonah, it could mean no more airport trips, big wire transfers, or fears of spoilage. Soon I learn that other Amish farmers are milking camels too: Noah in Pennsylvania, Dallas in Indiana, Clyde and Sam in Missouri. I order a few pints. After school, Jonah gets four ounces in his glass and doesn't know it's different. "Is it camel milk?"

"Yes, honey."

He drinks it without a fuss.

The Bedouin milk, precious as it is, tends to get a little sour over the fortnight that a bottle lasts us. Toward the end, Jonah makes faces and shudders. Tony saws the frozen plastic liter bottles in half with a bread knife so we can thaw less at a time. But the American milk comes in a smaller sixteen-ounce bottle and remains fresh longer.

Next day Jonah gets the same amount of the Amish camel milk. After a week, he's stable. After three weeks, he hasn't regressed. We return to the Bedouin milk and see no difference. "It works!" I rejoice. "It works."

Because this milk from a different continent also helps my son, we know the effect isn't dependent on the geographic source. It demonstrates that camel milk itself — not some magic herb in the Bedouin camels' diet or a special camel breed — is what helps Jonah. This "N of 1" experiment, as scientists call a single-person trial, means children in all countries may benefit from camel milk.

I hold a bottle of Amish milk to the sun. It doesn't look as powerful as the Bedouin milk, although I know this is speculation. I don't see those thick white globs around the rim, and it's thinner. But it seems to have the same benefits for Jonah, and that's good enough for me.

Now that we have a reliable supply, I can spread the news. It's time for me to share our camel milk miracle with the world.

13 A PUBLIC BIRTH

"You must be very patient."
— GIL RIEGLER

Before Christmas, I'm bent over my desk with notes and my "camel papers" — the books, articles, and copies of old journals I've collected, adding a touch of history to the article I've been writing for weeks. "Got [Camel] Milk?" explains what's special about camel milk, who's likely to benefit from it, and Jonah's story. It outlines why it's hard to transport the milk from remote deserts to towns. There's a photo of Gil and me grinning at baggage claim with suitcases of Bedouin milk he has just brought in.

Three months later, the article is online and going viral. A day after that, foreign websites chop it up and repurpose it in quirky English and other languages. Emails start flooding in. It's the most widely read piece I've ever written. I find myself communicating with scientists, veterinarians, and more parents.

In response to the increase in curiosity about camels, Gil and Nancy at Oasis are hosting the first US camel clinic. What topics are on the agenda for this unique event? Camel wrangling, milking, fertility, and more. I drive to Oasis to present my camel milk research and our story for the very first time. But it's not like my previous speaking events. The conference venue is a barnyard, and the stage is grassy dirt. The podium is a battered picnic table.

Never having been to a camel gathering, I expect grizzled cowboys in boots. There's just one, almost eighty, and he looks like a Western movie star but says nothing. His wife, pretty in her blonde-gray braids, wants to keep camels, and they've flown here to investigate. The trouble is, their place is on the Big Island in Hawaii, where the soil is sharp with volcanic glass, sand, and rock. Camels might cut their soft, padded feet, and what are they going to graze on?

The other men are camel guys, the good ol' boys of the exotic animal world. They're in work boots and tennis shoes, trucker hats, faded T-shirts over bulging bellies. There are women, too: ranchers in flannel shirts who pay the bills by exhibiting animals, luxury-home matriarchs with backyard menageries, ponytailed livestock wranglers, grandmas in gold earrings. Most of these folks already own animals; camels, goats, sheep, horses, and zebras. Many take their camels to Christmas Nativity scenes or to school events and fairs. They might breed and trade baby camels at auctions or online. They love all sorts of creatures — the more exotic, the better.

There is talk about Marlin Troyer, the surly Amish man I know from the Facebook camel milk group. I can't wait to meet him. But everyone's wondering, how will he get here if he doesn't drive a car? Soon I see a youngish man getting out of a black sedan. He wears a green shirt and pants and a matching green felt hat, like Robin Hood. He's not the classic Amish figure the camel people are expecting, but Danny, a Southern camel-ride operator, swears it's him.

"But he's not in a straw hat or black suit. And he's got a rental car," we say.

"He's a Amish. I knowed 'em all my life. I might be wrong about a buncha other things, but he's a Amish."

During the break, I gather the courage to approach Marlin. "Do you want to go to lunch?"

"I might." He takes his car, I take mine.

We sit at a picnic table in a wood-hewn café off the highway. I'm a little afraid of this ranting Facebook ogre, with his bad spelling and passionate rants. And I'm still wondering how an Amish person can go online like he does.

Over sandwiches he doesn't exactly apologize, but his suspicion lessens once he hears my son's story. His smile is infrequent yet charismatic. His trim form exudes a feeling of restrained wildness, as if he's wary of confinement. With his green eyes, springy hair, and beard, he's like an exotic cat.

"How did you travel here?"

"I flew. Got a rental car."

I imagine he's new to driving, but I don't really know. Is he still Amish? If he's some other religion now, he probably hasn't been for long. His accent is long and flat. There are cultural things he doesn't know, like references to music or other countries. It's like talking to a time traveler from seventy-five years ago.

After leaving the Old Order Amish, he's become an unaffiliated Mennonite, as some Amish do. He wanted to go online, and he rejected the High German spoken in his church services. To his mind, this language was an obstacle to sharing the gospel, since, he says, most Amish speak English. He's recently switched from a horse and buggy to a car, but he still lives largely by Amish-friendly principles.

Marlin first got camels two years ago, purchasing three from Sam Hostetler, an Amish farmer in Missouri who brokers exotic animals. "I've always been interested in exotics," he says. "Had some time and money free up after I sold my furniture business. I planned to buy a zebra." But he was drawn to camels instead. His first camels weren't 'bred,' so they didn't produce a baby. Then he bought a pregnant camel from a source in Oklahoma. His first baby camel was born eighteen months ago in a portable mini-barn pulled next to his bedroom window, so he could check on the mother and baby while sitting up in bed. He's the second American farmer to sell the milk for human consumption, the first being Noah Peachey in rural Pennsylvania.

Many states allow raw milk sales. But a tangle of regulations from the FDA and USDA effectively bans raw milk from crossing state lines. Marlin and some Amish farmers (and various dairy and legal experts) view the federal laws as unconstitutional. They would like the chance to sell both raw and pasteurized milk outside of their states, and they have discussed selling their milk through a membership club, "based on the right of private association as stated in the First and Fourteenth Amendments," he clarifies.

"It's cold up in Michigan in the winter," I remark. "How do the camels do?"

"They're just fine. I've got a barn for them. Only problem is when their feet get wet in the spring, they can get parasites. We're solving that one right now. As far as the milk, moms are calling me, thanking me. Crying in gratitude for their kids' improvements," he says. "Is that the kind of thing you saw with your son?"

"Yes, it is. I know the feeling," I say.

"I have never seen anything like that. I mean, the letters I get! I had heard it was good for autism, but I didn't expect this."

"And the other guys, are they seeing the same thing?"

"They are. It makes you thankful to serve the families. I've got a wife and three boys. Lucky for me my kids are fine."

"Do you use it at home too?"

"We sure do." He shakes his head slowly, his white teeth barely showing in a hint of a smile. "We are just blessed to do this work." He abruptly seems to make up his mind to accept me, declaring he's got to meet someone, but he'll see me later at the clinic. I think our meeting was a success.

Next day, there's a cadre of cashmere sweater wearers in tasteful shoes. Their Mercedes and BMWs shine in the swirling dust of the parking lot. They look like a highly polished get-rich-quick set.

"Where did these people come from?" I ask Gil.

"They've heard the news about camel milk. They're potential investors. They want to see how much money's in this. Some came from Beverly Hills and LA." After listening to a couple of talks, they're gone. They don't stay to learn about autism. They miss other good stuff, too: camel-handling lessons.

To keep such a large, strong, and willful animal you must be able to control it. Camels need a firm hand in their early training so they don't take over later. The camel's ability to kick out in every direction (there's no safe place around an irritated camel) means you have to be able to move it, rather than it moving you.

One of the most important skills is cushing — or kooshing, or hooshing, depending on what language the handler speaks. There seems to be no definitive spelling of the term — not a surprise considering that camels are mainly kept by nomads with oral, not written, traditions — but it's based on a variant of *coucher*, the French verb for lying down. Phrases differ: Arabs say "icckkkhh" or give a sharp, growling "hrrrrr." In the United States it's "cush," rhyming with *push*.

Teaching a camel to cush takes six steps: touching the legs; placing a rope around the left foreleg; holding the leg in a bent position with the rope and running it behind the hump (or between the humps, for a Bactrian camel) to the other side; gently pulling the camel down on its bent knee while saying "cush"; waiting for the rump to follow; then asking the camel to stand up again. These steps are repeated until the skill is learned. Gil and a helper bring a camel to show us how it's done.

The young male camel is in a halter, with Gil holding its rope. The other man loops a light rope around the camel's left front foot. This handling is all new to a young camel, especially if it's a bottle-fed baby, bought young and not raised with a herd. This camel seems very calm, but when the helper twitches the rope, just to get him accustomed to its movement, he gets antsy, like there's a tag in his T-shirt.

"Good boy," Gil says soothingly.

The rope pulls tighter, and the camel gives a low, rumbly moo. He shifts his backside in a circle around Gil. He knows there's a grain bucket in his future, but how can he get it?

Gil picks up a long, thin rod and tickles him with the handle, offering a pleasant scratch. The camel makes comfortable "uhuhuh" sounds. "He's still talking to me," Gil says. "That shows he's okay." The other man pulls the rope up, bending the camel's leg at the knee. The camel flails, but his free leg takes the weight. The helper loops the rope behind the hump, walking around the camel's rear. The camel spots the grain by the fence.

"Cush, cush, cush," coaxes Gil. The camel shifts and stumbles. His free knee drops, and down he goes. But he resists, trying to stand on his hobbled foot like an amputee. Up he rises.

"Cush, you're okay, you're okay, good boy," says Gil, tickling his free foot with the rod. It takes a whole minute before the other front leg bends. The camel is half-down, but the rest of him must follow. Gil tickles his back foot. They're in a stalemate; then the camel's ears twitch, a sign he's going down. His back legs fold like a hinge. "Good boy!"

"He's not stressed or nervous," Gil says. Camels express stress through their poop, which looks like food: peanuts, grapes, and guacamole. Peanuts mean no or slight stress, grapes mean "I don't like this," and "blowing guacamole" means "I'm done."

The process can be just as stressful for the trainer as for the camel. "You must be very patient," says Gil. "Once you start a training session, you can't stop till the end." Normally he would take more time with the camel, he says, but this session is accelerated for the audience.

Gil's training method is basic behaviorism in action. He offers something the animal wants, called a reinforcer (the grain), gives the instruction (the command to cush), and prompts the camel to do the behavior (stimulating and lifting the leg). He's verbally encouraging (offering soothing comments), he breaks the tasks into small sections (giving a rest between stages), and then gives praise and the reinforcer when the task is done. He'll gradually reduce the prompts and reinforcers as the task is mastered.

Standing upright again, the camel munches his grain, lips sliding sideways over jutting lower teeth. He's as calm as a baby. Gil kisses his nose. All these people kiss their camels, like giving a blessing or in a joyful outburst. Facebook photos from almost every country show human lips pressed on camel noses, men and women alike. Having well-trained camels makes everyone glow.

Why do camels need to be trained? People who don't train their camels properly and can't handle them usually get rid of them. They go to people like Gil and Nancy, who end up running a camel foster home of sorts. They calm the animals, teach them, give them a role. And training enables them to work. Working camels live longer than those who don't work, say experts. Learning and socialization isn't bad for them — they're social creatures, and their health is at risk if they can't contribute to a group or interact with others. (This is a challenge shared by people with significant mental and emotional problems, prisoners, and those whose behavior impairs their social skills.)

After the lesson I'm scheduled to speak about camel milk, but a camel guy rushes up. "Your talk is delayed. Come out to the field!" I walk through the brush, bright in the afternoon sun, to join a crowd waiting by an open shed.

Dr. Ahmed Tibary is standing over a pregnant camel lying on the ground. Tall, with thick dark hair and eyebrows, he's a top camel-fertility vet. This mother couldn't have a better midwife. Soon a head slithers from her birth canal, gray and wet. A long foreleg follows. Tibary tugs on it but cautions, "We cannot rush her. She isn't that dilated."

The camel can't see what's going on but lies patiently, noiselessly, as more of the leg emerges. Tibary wipes the calf's mouth.

He's deft and focused. His experience has included performing up to seven camel C-sections in a day and implanting thousands of embryos in Middle Eastern breeding camels. He tugs again, and the camel pudenda, if there is such a thing, protrudes like a large, furry belly button. The baby seems stuck. Tibary pulls both forelegs, easing its shoulders out. The mother camel rises, and the baby is born, falling backward and landing with its neck folded against its head. Such a delivery would break a normal creature, but the baby lifts its pointy gray head, jerking in fits and starts.

Tibary peels a thin white caul, like dried glue, from the baby's face and body. Its neck flops like a snake. Two minutes later it rolls itself upright onto its bulging knees.

The mother placidly noses it for a few seconds but then seems to dismiss it, like she's saying, "It's time for my nap. Turn on the TV if you get bored."

The big question is the sex of this spindly creature, which spells its destiny: fearsome bull, gelded workman, queen mother? Contrary to the norms of most human societies, female camels are prized over males.

"Gil always calls it a boy before it's born, hoping not to be disappointed," says Nancy, shooting a video of the birth from the shed's rails.

"It's a boy," murmurs Tibary.

"Aw, well. Boys are good too," says Nancy.

Tibary wipes the baby's muzzle with water. A second glimpse of the baby's underside reveals a better view. "It's a girl!" he says.

"What should we name her?" Nancy asks the buzzing crowd.

"Name her Tibaria," calls someone.

"How about Maya?" says a woman with a yoga-soft voice.

The baby struggles to rise. Soon she's standing, fluffy as an Easter lamb. Her legs splay like wobbly tent poles braced against the wind of the world. Golden rays of sunshine sweep the shed, the first light that has ever touched her eyes. What does she see, smell, taste, and think?

Her name, Gil decides, is Luna. With the birth over, we all rush to the picnic table, and as birds squawk loudly in the trees overhead, I begin my talk.

During my presentation, the tree-shaded computer screen illustrates my son's case. I lay out his history, his symptoms, and the course of his improvement. I explain the unique properties of the camel's oval blood cells and antibodies and discuss the new studies I've found. I highlight the milk's enzymes and its antiviral, antibacterial properties. I explain the connections between autism and immune response and the reasons why camel milk may help with the behavioral and physical problems associated with autism. I list other health conditions it might mitigate: ADHD, food allergies, Crohn's disease, Machado-Joseph disease (a dire neurological disorder), skin conditions, liver disease, hepatitis, tuberculosis. I share the challenges in dealing with the USDA, which basically discourages camel importation (a hope I've given up). I mention the FDA's long-standing disinterest in natural therapies. I end with the problems faced by customers and milk sellers in developing countries, where camel owners don't have refrigerated delivery, and nomads haul milk jugs on motorbikes.

When it's over, one by one, three sturdy camel handlers approach. Does it sound like my child has autism? they ask. I outline recommended diets, give advice on schooling, suggest therapies, lend a sympathetic ear.

As the sun sinks lower over the fields, a Middle Eastern–style feast is set out. Darkness falls, a banjo appears, and cameleers sing and tell stories. The humor and teasing reveal their camaraderie. If you love camels, you join a community that will help you without question. When I came here with my strange story about camel milk, they never blinked an eye. Since I first found out about it, I've wanted to help autism families get the milk, and my interest in camels keeps growing. Today has shown how the two subjects work in tandem, making the world better for humans and animals.

14 CAMEL FEEL THE SOUL

"Camel can feel and attack."
— Dr. Abdul Raziq Kakar

Every camel culture is different, but they all share a truth: camels have a prodigious memory. Their ability to love and hate is legendary, their attachments like iron. They mourn deceased owners, respond to music, work harder when sung to by Bedouins. Their minds, say some cameleers, resemble those of human children; some speculate that among nonhuman mammals, they are second in intelligence only to dogs (although the human perception of animal intelligence is highly skewed by our perspective). Given their innate preference for doing things their way, camels' smarts make them tricky to handle.

People ask me if I own camels. I don't have the will or the space to handle even one. To manage a camel, a person must speak its language. The camel must trust its handler if it is to obey and give milk. Owners who don't live side by side with camels must hire a camel nanny of sorts, to sweet-talk, train, feed, restrain, medicate, and observe the animals.

Not only are camels smart and resourceful, but they have no natural predators (although starving animals such as wolves may attack dromedaries, and wild Bactrians have some foes and are more flight-prone). Thanks to their position atop the food chain in their native lands, they don't panic easily and are hard to intimidate. If someone angers them, they'll crush him, or sit on his head like it was a cheap lawn chair, tearing the guts from anyone who interferes. Cruelty to a camel is a boomerang for the owner, returning when he least expects it.

Ever hear the phrase "She bit my head off"? A drunk man in India met a camel tied near a footpath. Something disagreeable occurred, and it *did* bite his head off. Then the camel — a male — tore the leg from a bystander who tried to help. A week later, when blood tests at the animal shelter verified that the camel was perfectly healthy and not rabid, the owner led him home. On the way, the camel severed his arm at the elbow. Back the camel went for more tests. But the locals already knew. "If he wanted to breed and had a memory of it, and there was no girl camel around, he can get angry and bite," one said. They don't need tests. They know camels.

Camels' heads pivot all the way around, and their powerful legs can kick you into the grave. They can swing a man in their teeth like a rag doll. But their preferred method of killing is simply crushing opponents to death. An American camel farmer showed me a picture of the remnants of a wheelbarrow flattened like a piece of toast by a camel that jumped out of a horse stall. Luckily the farmer leapt out of the way.

Sure, cattle can be dangerous too, especially bulls. My dad told us once to stay away from the bull on our Appalachian farm. But I waded the creek on an errand and saw him alone in his pasture. His head turned to me, stolid and mountainous, like a heavyweight fighter with a concussion. I wondered briefly at my dad's wisdom in using only our painfully unpredictable electric fence to contain this bull. But he just twitched an ear as I edged through the weeds. Camel owners have a confident streak much like my dad's. Optimism is buying an animal that can grow to weigh two tons.

Camels impress me with their physical bigness, no matter how often I'm around them. Usually calm, they're also nimble, and while I've never had a problem, there's a risk of getting shoved, stepped on, or sat on, even if they're in a good mood. Take the fourteen camels I visited in Noah's barn in Pennsylvania. The cute, snow-white babies stared at me hesitantly, and I longed to touch their soft curly hair. The big ones ignored me, and the teenagers slobbered on my coat sleeve for attention. Though they were fenced, fed, and content, being at such close quarters with them still kept me vigilant. They can't help it, they're just *large*. Their unpredictable necks conjure an octopus's twisting grace.

These creatures are alluring at any age. At birth, the stilt-legged babies look as if they've been pulled from a flood, but they soon fluff up like a precious plush toy. Up to a year old, they're still leaning on mom but developing the skills for independence. At two or three years old they are playful "preschoolers." They kiss humans' faces, press eyelash to eyelash, hang their heads over people's arms. They may shy at fluttering ribbons and other alarming menaces, still adjusting to the world. By age four, they've achieved more self-confidence. While camels can be trained without special preparation once they're ready (ask a Bedouin), American owners of young "pet" camels might place blankets on their backs to accustom them to burdens. By six they're considered mature, ready to give rides, pull carts, and do a camel's work.

Camel mothers stand patiently, accommodating their babies' needs like all mothers do. They try to eat grass or hay with kids clinging to their bellies or snort off to a quiet corner when they've had enough. Female camels don't have a regular estrus cycle. They go into a bloodless three- to four-day "heat" (when they can get pregnant) every twenty-eight days or so, but only during the bulls' winter breeding season. Somewhat high-strung and sensitive when in heat, she-camels get restless and isolate themselves from the herd. They spray urine freely, spreading it with their tails, sometimes even mounting other females. They ovulate "on demand," releasing eggs like a vending machine once rutting bulls deposit their seed, which stimulates the females' reproductive hormones.

Other things can make camels irritable, too. One pregnant camel was so annoyed by her female owner's presence that she shoved her big head through a fence and attempted a double mastectomy with her teeth. "After she gave birth the next day, we both acted as if nothing happened," reports the owner. A wrist brace worn by another owner provoked months of alarm in her baby camel. In repeated attempts to "rescue" mom from the creature apparently eating her arm, the baby learned to undo the Velcro with her mouth.

Gelded male camels, the hardworking castrati of the herd, are often pretty calm. Their aggressive behavior is reduced by castration. Some think young camels are the most dangerous of them all because their size is coupled with a lack of maturity. "If not taught respect for personal space, animals can hurt humans when playing is allowed," says one veteran handler.

But bulls are petrifying. It takes a firm hand and a sense of mastery to handle a bull. They're as solid as a mountain and tall as a train car, with the strength of a dozen or more men. And they're born to breed and control. Getting between them and their desires can be fatal. And sometimes their reactions are personal.

"Camel feel the soul," writes Dr. Abdul Raziq Kakar, a respected Pakistani veterinarian and animal advocate I've met on Facebook. (Camel milk healed his arthritis, he reports, a sudden form so severe he could no longer walk.) "Male camel goes very sad and offensive sometime, especially when he is in rut and someone punish or hurt him. He can get very lonely in breeding season's short days and cold weather. If someone has bad intention or do not like him, camel can feel and attack."

Stories of dangerous camels abound. An Australian woman received a ten-month-old camel as a birthday gift from her husband. It reportedly straddled her in a misguided mating attempt. The camel was found wandering in the backyard while she lay dead nearby. A woman from Kazakhstan was killed by a camel she'd raised from infancy. Neighbors blamed the craziness of males in mating season. A man in Mexico was kicked, bitten, and smothered by a camel from his animal sanctuary. The camel was so angry it had to be pulled off his body by a truck. The locals think the camel was mad because his owner hadn't given him his usual Coca-Cola that day.

Even well-intentioned acts by humans can develop camels' aggression. Offering a big rubber ball for a camel to kick around the yard and capture under its chest sounds fun, but it teaches the camel how to press someone to death.

Fortunately, there's an online group for cameleers, where well-intentioned new owners can get help from old hands. Veterans like Gil repeat the advice born of long experience. A camel does not need "enrichment": it needs open fields, salt, other camels for company, green things to nibble, and that's about it. "Stop trying to make it human," they say, with occasional frustration (except Gil, who is preternaturally patient). Yet they welcome the novices and continue to share their knowledge. These delicate animals can't be treated like cattle or horses. Certain medicines can tear their guts; certain foods can kill them. There is no such thing as a stupid question about camels.

One thing becomes clear about camels: whether you have one camel or a thousand, they evoke both reverence and aggravation. Each camel has a unique personality and uncanny intelligence. Camel owners must never assume they have the upper hand, because the human advantage can disappear without warning. Your puny bag of bones will never be a match for a camel. Only the camel's love and tolerance allow you to survive. So you must earn your camel's respect with affection, firm boundaries, good care, and deep kindness.

15 THE POWER OF CAMEL MILK

"When my son gets in trouble, people go to the *hospital.*"
— MOTHER OF A SEVEN-YEAR-OLD BOY WITH AUTISM

I'm scheduled to give a talk about camel milk at a national autism conference. The organizers, who know my story, let Marlin bring camels to the parking lot. The kids with autism visit them, some fearlessly walking too close, with others slightly cowering, as they would from any animal. Parents probe Marlin about his feeding and milking practices, wanting to be sure their sensitive kids aren't exposed to allergens. In his hat and shirtsleeves, Marlin's beaming like a little boy. White-bearded church deacon Sam Hostetler, an Amish entrepreneur and growing camel milk producer, lends a pastoral presence with his knowledgeable grandmotherly wife. Sharing a booth with Clyde, another Amish camel farmer, they hand out brochures to people who want to buy their milk.

On the podium, I outline Jonah's story, give background on camels and their unique attributes, and share what I know about the science behind camel milk's effectiveness. It's similar to my camel clinic presentation but more tailored to parents.

The most important research I have to share is breaking news from Dr. Laila Al-Ayadhi, a researcher in Saudi Arabia. She's just done a double-blinded, randomized clinical trial using camel milk with sixty kids with autism. Oxidative stress, a biochemical imbalance associated with autism, decreased after the kids drank camel milk, and the severity of their symptoms dropped, as measured on the Childhood Autism Rating Scale (CARS). Patients with allergic-response issues were most likely to show improvement, a conclusion that matches my own.

Of course, I don't say that camel milk can *cure* autism. There's no cure (yet, if ever), although, given enough therapies and plain old luck, some kids lose most of their disabling symptoms. And there are worries about losing the often-valuable traits of honesty, dogged focus, intelligence, and pattern recognition that are heightened in some forms of autism. You'd never want to be ableist and have everyone conform to a standard. But treating the pain and impairments of autism is important.

Afterward, two mothers who've been nodding excitedly come up. One's using the milk already.

"My son was giving me problems. School was a big issue," she said, her deep brown eyes glowing with enthusiasm.

"Like you got calls to pick him up?"

"I wish. When my son gets in trouble, people go to the *hospital*."

I nod, imagining a big teen.

"How old is he?"

"Seven." Her friend nods sagely.

"He bit me so hard I had like thirty stitches right here," the mom says, grabbing her inner thigh to show me. "He hit his head on the wall so much the hair on his head rubbed off."

Even after my twelve years of autism work, I'm kind of speechless at this. "But I gave him the camel's milk and it stopped," she says.

"What stopped?"

"His aggression. And his hair grew back in."

"Any social things?"

She smiles. "He noticed his sister for the first time. I drive my kids to school, and he never interacted with her. But one day I said something silly, and I saw in the mirror that he actually looked at his sister, and connected with her eyes, like he was saying, 'Isn't Mom funny?'"

"He's a different kid," says her friend. "I can see the changes. I want to try it too."

"You have a child with autism?"

"Two," she says. Both of these mothers are black, another reason it's great to see them here. On average, black kids with autism are diagnosed years later than white kids, and many don't get early intervention.

Two more black women approach. Their accents and long dresses turn out to be Kenyan. "My son is doing well on camel milk already. He's in Kenya now," says one, serene and confident.

"I'm going to bring my son there soon so he can drink it too," says the other.

I have conversations like this throughout the conference. They continue long after it's over. Everyone I tell about camel milk wants to know, Why does it work? There are no definitive answers, but here are some hypotheses based on recent research.

Even a few years ago, doctors might have scoffed at the idea that autism, long seen as a neurological or psychiatric disorder, could be linked to the immune system, let alone to the health of the gut. But today's medical researchers are interested in immune response and the "microbiome" — the vast population of bacteria and other microbes that inhabit the human body, particularly the gut. Evidence is emerging that the composition of the microbiome may significantly influence our physical and mental health. Some of our resident bacteria are beneficial, and help us digest food and nutrients. Others are potentially harmful — and the ways our immune system tries to eliminate them can be damaging.

Inflammation is a powerful emergency response mounted by the immune system to fight infection. It happens normally in fever, or when a burn or cut needs healing. But a prolonged immune response releases chemicals that can harm the body and brain. Such long-term inflammation prevents the immune system from working normally. It may be a factor in several diseases, including diabetes, Crohn's, colitis, rheumatoid arthritis, eczema, and autism (all of which are often treated with dietary modifications).

The connection of inflammation to autism is becoming more clearly established. Pregnant women with inflammatory conditions (including diabetes, preeclampsia, bacterial infections, and asthma) may be more likely to have a baby with autism. Children with autism have decreased immune system regulation. Different types of autism are linked to gut bacteria that can alter immune response as well as result in autistic behavior. A study of autistic children with gastrointestinal (GI) issues shows unusual levels of the proteins that regulate the permeability of the gut. Gut wall dysfunction can create what is often called "leaky gut" syndrome. This allows bacteria, undigested food particles, and toxins to enter the bloodstream. If these substances cross the blood-brain barrier, they may cause deficits in neurological functioning. Those without GI symptoms may have other forms of inflammation.

So what is it about camel milk that can boost gut health and the immune system and reduce both the GI and behavioral symptoms associated with autism? There is much that we still don't understand, but the more likely factors can be noted.

Camel milk contains essential fatty acids, a high level of insulin (or a similar protein), vitamins, and minerals, which may account for some of its benefits. The most important components of camel milk, though, may be its unique enzymes, immunoglobulins, and other proteins.

Three significant enzymes are lysozyme, an enzyme that can destroy bacterial cell walls, mitigate food allergies, and help repair compromised immune systems; lactoperoxidase, found in all animal milk, tears, and saliva, which boosts antiviral and antibacterial activity, promotes growth, and may fight tumors; and the enzyme NAGase, which is antibacterial and similar to enzymes found in human breast milk.

Camel milk's powerful proteins have been credited with immunological, antioxidant, and anticancer effects. Lactoferrin can combat the growth of harmful gut microbes that may be partly responsible for the digestive problems commonly experienced by autistic children. When camel milk is ingested, it may produce peptides (small chains of amino acids, the components of proteins) that act as natural antioxidants and combat conditions associated with oxidative stress. Children with autism-related immune-system deficits have a decreased ability to process free radicals (toxic byproducts of our metabolism), which leads to oxidative stress. The brain is highly sensitive to oxidative stress, and camel milk's proteins and nutrients may reduce its effects by regulating inflammatory pathways.

The milk may also induce a calming effect by regulating levels of the neurotransmitters dopamine and serotonin. Neurotransmitters are chemicals that transmit signals in the nervous system. GABA (gamma-aminobutyric acid), a neurotransmitter that lowers brain and central nervous system activity, is found in high levels in camel milk, and it may work its effects on the brain when it's absorbed through the gut.

Camel milk also contains natural probiotics — beneficial gut bacteria — as well as higher quantities of the nutrients that support the body's own population of beneficial bacteria. (Commercial probiotic supplements are heavily marketed to autism families.) There is evidence that some children with autism lack several strains of beneficial gut bacteria. These are important because they break down chemicals in food that can cause adverse digestive and behavioral effects.

Like all animal milks, camel milk contains immunoglobulins (IgGs), or antibodies, from the mothers' immune system. These enable baby animals to resist infection before they can produce their own antibodies. The immunoglobulins produced by camels are tiny, one-half to one-tenth the size of humans'. This enables them to penetrate and kill bacteria and viruses better than other IgGs. (Their increased effectiveness may be one reason why camels are resistant to some common animal diseases.)

These small IgG molecules are encapsulated in structures called micelles. The micelles may protect the IgGs from digestive enzymes in the gastrointestinal tract and help keep them intact for absorption into the blood stream. (Camel milk proteins may have other traits that prevent absorption.) Camel micelles are larger and more stable than those in cow milk, so it's likely that more IgGs remain intact to be delivered to cells throughout the body. Mothers who drink camel milk while nursing and give it to their children say that their children's rashes, food intolerances, nutritional malabsorption, and failure to gain weight are largely resolved. These results likely stem from improved immune response and healing of the "leaky gut." Some adults with severe digestive issues also report improvements with use of camel milk. (The lactose in camel milk differs from that of cow milk and is well accepted by most lactose-intolerant people.)

All animal milks are laden with healthy substances to nourish growing babies, so why is it that cow milk doesn't have the same benefits in reducing autism symptoms, and often actually aggravates them? One problem may lie with casein, a protein found in all mammary milk but more abundant in cow milk. It has several subtypes, but the one known as A1 beta-casein may worsen autism. When digested, it can form beta-casomorphin-7, an opioid peptide that may escape the leaky gut, pass the blood-brain barrier, and aggravate behavioral symptoms such as detachment, lack of interest in exploring one's surroundings, and lowered social interaction. And the casein in camel milk also differs from cow milk casein and rarely causes problems in cow milk–allergic kids.

Every child is different, and published research may not address highly individualized responses to diet. It is still difficult to know whether any dietary interventions, or what kind, will work for a child. Sometimes there are physical indications of food intolerances, like rashes, yeast, red cheeks, bumps, and under-eye circles. These are sometimes accompanied by a family history of inflammation-related disorders, dietary issues, and autism-spectrum characteristics. But some kids who don't exhibit these physical signs improve on camel milk anyway.

For Jonah, dairy protein in all forms — organic or regular milk, cheese, casein, milk powder, whey, and even goat milk — clearly had an adverse effect. Within three weeks of removing it from his diet when he was almost three, his language began to return and his unusual behaviors decreased. But for him, camel milk is more than just a nonallergenic substitute for cow milk: it has led to significant improvements in his physical well-being and behavior.

So if camel milk is so great, why hasn't the FDA approved it for treating autism? It's accepted as a healthy and legal food, but claiming that it has medical benefits requires compiling an FDA submission with the scientific evidence to substantiate it. Developing that evidence (through studies or clinical trials) is an expensive and lengthy process. There's little business incentive for a company to pursue approval of claims for camel milk, since, even if they succeeded, they could not control consumers' access to the milk. Sure, a company could try to identify and patent the effective components, then create a protected drug. That route, however, would require millions of dollars for the clinical trials, and they'd lose the money if a competitor succeeded first. Even then, another company could slightly alter the formula and make a knock-off version.

Still, marketing a drug is the quintessentially American solution to illness. Many people who wouldn't touch camel milk would readily swallow a pill. I hope someone makes camel milk a "nutraceutical" or a drug. It would be far easier, if not as entertaining, to call in an order to the local pharmacy. But a drug derived from camel milk would doubtless be expensive — and might lose something precious in the process.

In the meantime, word has been getting around about the benefits of camel milk. In Indiana, Colorado, Michigan, Missouri, and Pennsylvania, camel farmers have been inundated with requests. Most customers become regulars, getting cases of pint bottles in cold boxes. When I mention it to a local businessman, he tells me his nineteen-year-old severely autistic son just started drinking it. This kind of autism often comes with bowel problems. Tall and nonverbal, the son has just had the first formed stools of his life. When you think about changing a grown man's messy diaper, that's a pretty significant plus.

The bottom line is, this milk is worthy of protection. From desert to city, camel nomads are being proven right. Their treasured ancient pharmacy deserves new recognition.

16 THE AMISH TAKE CAMELS ON FAITH

"It will happen if the good Lord's plan is so."
— BEN, AMISH FARMER

The town of Bird-in-Hand has camels in barns. They live on the farm of the Miller brothers. Bird-in-Hand, one of many quaintly named Pennsylvania Dutch towns, lies at the western tip of a triangle formed with Gap and Blue Ball. Since I'm visiting Philadelphia with Tony, I can visit the farm. I might get a bottle or send customers here, so I want to see how it's run.

Leaving downtown Philly, I skirt the suburban big-box stores. The landscape softens into old roads and settled towns. Green lawns zing with the sound of summer bugs. It feels like horse-drawn carriages are clip-clopping just ahead.

Nearly two hours later, I'm not just lost, I'm country lost. Every turn looks the same, all the roads lined with green fields and pristine barns. Amish women in shape-hiding dresses of blue and soft earth tones drive horse-drawn buggies over the blacktop. Boys dressed as little men, young girls in white caps, and women skim along on bicycles. But when I look closer, I see they're not pedaling. They stand with one foot on flat running boards between the wheels, the other foot pushing them forward. The bikes move fast despite their lack of gears. From a distance, they show smooth and constant purpose.

I'm looking for Miller's farm because Noah Peachey, an Amish camel farmer I've helped with a brochure, sent me here. Noah's place, called Drome-Dairy, is one or two hours farther out, depending on who I ask, so I'll head his way later. These farmers offer sketchy details of car travel times. If I'd asked about driving a buggy, I'd probably get a great estimate — "Mebbe a day and a half," they might say. And my cellphone is confused by this rural location. So I'm stuck in a loop.

I'm tempted to call the Millers, but I hate to intrude. Even if Amish folks now have access to cellphones and fax machines, these technologies just aren't their way. Sam Hostetler, of Missouri's Humpback Dairy, has sent me a scant text or two. Noah uses a phone for two hours a day; Dallas of Indiana can schedule a call with a week's notice. Amish farmers may have a website but not use it directly, like the Millers (who do record their own voicemail greeting). Farmers like them often employ intermediaries to manage their email and computer work.

I give up and call. An unruffled man answers and directs me to the farm.

In a quiet patch of dirt, I pull over, open the car door, and slide down in the seat, wiggling from my shorts and tank top into jeans and a shirt. It's hot, but I don't want to show up with bare legs and shoulders. "English" (non-Amish) people like me aren't expected to dress "plainly." But Amish women avoid makeup or jewelry. So, out of respect, I'm doing the same.

I pull up near a white house on a typical farm driveway and park behind a buggy with steel wheels. Rubberless wheels might be the sign of a very conservative Amish order.

An Amish man is leaning over a curly-corded telephone in a homemade phone booth outside a building. I scuff my shoe in the gravel to alert him.

An older man with graying hair under his flat-brimmed straw hat comes over. "Are you looking for someone?"

"Yes, Amos Miller."

"That would be him in there. So are you Christina? I heard that name."

"Yes, I'm a writer, and I write about camel milk. My son has benefited from drinking it."

His face changes pretty quickly when he hears *writer*, and he seems to move his body away and turn at the same time, still friendly but more guarded. "Okay, he'll be there in a minute," he says briskly, then leaves. Amos ends his call, gets up, and turns around.

In our two phone conversations he's been formal and soft-spoken, giving the impression of a family patriarch. But Marlin had told me the Millers were young brothers with many kids. Amos is young, fair-skinned, and light-eyed, with a long beard and suspenders. He resembles the photos of my Civil War ancestors.

"Hello," he says, the O dipping into a slide. "You're that camel lady." He smiles at me, although not much.

"That would be me." I don't extend my hand, as I'm unsure of his rules.

"I got about an hour for ya today. I wanted to give ya more, but I got things to do. You want to see the operation?"

"Sure I do."

"Come on this way," he says, friendly but formal. Business is still on his mind. "I can't stay too long, but then you can talk to the other guys." I follow him to the building, an unremarkable packing shed.

Inside is the large and multifaceted home of Miller's Organic Farm. First, there's a smell of milk and blood. Passing two young boys sealing raw chicken parts into vacuum bags, we enter the cold-storage room. Jars of pickled and savory foods fill the wooden shelves. But mostly I see blocks of cheese: aged dill and onion, pepper jack, cheddar, all kinds, in shades of mustard, almond, and cream. There are dozens of prepared foods, and I catch a glimpse of the meats in back. I'm filling imaginary picnic baskets and planning barbecues. Shredded carrots, tomatoes, kombucha — almost anything, it seems, can be jarred. Fermented ketchup: "Tomato paste, fish sauce, maple syrup, whey, garlic, Celtic sea salt, cayenne pepper," reads the label. I imagine women and children chopping and pouring for days, from recipes shared after worship or at weddings.

A metal bucket in the far corner brims with brown liquid, rich with yellow bubbles. It's fresh chicken broth waiting to be packaged.

Amos half-turns his head and cautions, "Now we go into the meat area. Some people are bothered by this."

We pass two carcasses of mutton and beef hung up for cutting. "I'm not. I lived on a farm."

Amos says, "Back here is the killing place, where we shoot the animals. Some people are bothered by that."

On hog-killing days my dad kept us girls in the kitchen, hand-cranking pork scraps through a black iron sausage grinder. Fresh-spiced pork sizzling in a cast-iron skillet can't be gained without sacrifice. "I'm not," I say again.

In the back of the shed, a young guy adjusts a newly decapitated cow to hang just so on a rail. Bits of flesh sprinkle the floor. Now I see why some people are bothered.

Outside, a few stinking hides swarm with flies. I wade through the grass toward a weathered wooden pen, to see two new litters of baby pigs with doglike eyes.

Amos's desk in the shed is just a wooden shelf — no phone, no computer. He's holding a thick sheaf of papers. Curled at the edges from years of handling, it bears names and addresses both typed and handwritten. Miller's Organic ships close to $3 million worth of food a year, with pallets going regularly to New York, Florida, and California. Grass-fed beef, lamb, and mutton. Tons of cheese. Bags of potato chips and nuts, processed with an eye toward organic guidelines and those of the ancestral-diet advocate Dr. Weston A. Price. They've got a hefty base of customers far from Lancaster County.

Amos has heard from more customers looking for camel milk. "I got a lot of interest in the product in March," he says, although he doesn't seem to know that this spike may have been due to my "Got [Camel] Milk?" article. They got another surge in orders from parents after the autism conference where Sam and Marlin brought their camels to the parking lot. Any article or talk about camel milk increases sales for all the merchants.

"As of today, I have over two hundred camel milk customers in the membership." He seems bemused. "At first I didn't know if it was a good idea."

"Ben had the idea we should get camels," Amos says. "You should talk to him. And Samuel is the handler." Samuel lives a few acres away. I offer Amos a ride, but he prefers to take his push-bike, sailing down the hill and up the other side. Driving slowly, savoring the fields and open sky, I pass two boys on push-bikes. Amos moves fast, arriving the same time as I do. I get out of the car and see a herd of sand-brown camels standing in emerald-green pasture. Until now, I've only seen them against the stark dry hills of Southern California. I'm stricken with camelid cognitive dissonance.

Samuel, a smaller, blonder version of Amos, is a man of even fewer words. Ben is here too, a tall, dark-haired man with black glasses. Both have bowl haircuts and beards. Samuel, preferring action to speech, goes to fetch the camels for milking.

Around the corner comes one big camel, followed by others of different sizes. They roam, circle, or stand patiently, with movements more fluid than those of horses or cows. Although they're standoffish, they're curious about me. Flexible necks are prying in my business. Lips reach for my sleeve. A whiskered nose pokes my face. The babies are extra friendly. The white one stares at me through long lashes, like a living plush toy.

This milking barn, formerly used for cows, holds three stalls. The camels come in for milking or in bad weather, as some dislike the rain. They seem content, with an underlying eagerness to be milked. The rustling of the hay as they move through the barn and their crisp munching sounds, so soft on the ear, are cozily domestic. They look out of place but seem to feel right at home.

Samuel's sense of belonging among the animals is almost palpable. He moves among them as if entranced, but with the ease of the familiar. But while other camel owners enjoy the novelty of their origin, he, like most Amish, seems to view them as just another farm animal.

It's time for milking. "Wanna help?" asks Samuel. Using sounds and very few words, he leads each one toward the milking stalls. As a camel turns the corner, I clip its lead to a bar. Leaning under each large head is scary, but it's exciting to see the row of thick, arched necks lined up for milking. Samuel wipes the teats with a cloth. The baby camel nuzzles the first mother camel as Samuel attaches vacuum tubes to her teats. The tubes connect to a small milking machine resembling a tea-kettle, powered by a diesel line from the barn.

Camel milk comes fast. The camel stands still and content as her milk lets down and rushes through the clear tubes attached to her udder, her body stiff and quiet, her eyelids half-closed with the influx of nursing hormones. The baby camel shuffles nervously, looking for his share, but the mother ignores him completely.

"Can I take a picture of the milking?" I ask.

"You can take a picture of anything, just not of people," he says.

"No problem," I say. I'm glad he's not awkward, because I'm try-ing hard not to give offense. Like the camels, I'm not native to this part of the world — but then again, neither are the Amish.

The flow of milk subsides into froth. Samuel takes the tubes off. "Three minutes!" I say. That's double the time desert camels are said to take. But we're not in a sandstorm or sub-Saharan temperatures, so maybe it's an unfair comparison. They're averaging one hundred ounces of milk a day per camel   six to seven 16-ounce bottles, Amos says. The baby comes up and snuffles for milk. I feel a bit guilty, but the young camels get plenty at other times.

"Welcome to the zoo," says a sign above the milk room. Samuel brings the fresh warm milk inside and empties it into a metal bowl, strains it into a pitcher, and then tips it into pint bottles. He sets them in an old-fashioned cooler, rimmed with ice crystals, which is chilled by a diesel engine. This setup is so ingenious I'd never have known that it wasn't electrical.

Something else is different from the barns I'm used to. It has the scent of sawdust. "It's cleaner, not as smelly as cow barns," I say, and Samuel nods.

Ben turns out to be a talker by Amish standards. He tells me he got the idea for camels from Noah, and describes their feed. "We use grass with a little non-GMO grain. That's what the customers want. We put them on pasture in the summer. They're milking pretty good each day." He leans against a pole, looking relaxed. Ben has significant experience with the "English" world. This is partly thanks to little John, who's looking up at his daddy.

"Hey there! I like your backpack," I say. Black and small, it looks cute but not quite Amish.

"That's what he keeps his equipment in. He can't eat. He gets synthetic formula pumped through a feeding tube," says Ben. John, it turns out, not only has type 1 diabetes but has also had a bone marrow and a liver transplant. Since then, the family has endured battles with the hospital over John's diet and treatment.

"Was he drinking camel milk?" I ask.

"Yes, he was doing well on it." Temporary doctors who didn't know the family were spooked and stopped it, Ben says, but it had helped John gain weight. "The regular doctor restored the milk. He drinks it again now, and he's better. We've learned it's the closest to a natural medicine needed to prevent liver rejection. When we try to do without it, his liver enzyme numbers can skyrocket."

Looking small for his age, which is seven, this darling little man wears the straw hat, black suspenders, and coat of his older kin and has a huge smile on his freckled face. As a special-needs mom, I can't help but wonder what will happen when it's his time to wed. The Amish choose their own partners; marriages are not arranged, and I hope his illness won't cause rejection. Is this connect-the-dots community more accepting of disability than we English? Perhaps a tight-knit world is better in some ways. If I'd found a community like this to accept my son, I'd have turned Amish in a minute. But they don't seek converts, and those who try mostly fail. It's not the manual labor that challenges them so much as accepting the rigorous faith brought from Europe hundreds of years ago.

In the corner Samuel's little blonde daughter clasps a lanky barn cat around the ribs, its legs straight out in the air. The big cat stays limp. Her handmade brown dress and sturdy bare feet highlight her beaming, pink-cheeked face. Only two years old, she shares her joy, repeating a few phrases in the German dialect called Pennsylvania Dutch. I don't know what she means, and she doesn't understand me, so all I can do is smile. Amish kids learn English once they start school, which stops at eighth grade. And the language of their religion is often High German, so she'll be trilingual in a way.

Nearby, her preschool-aged brother competently carries a bucket. Samuel speaks to him, and he goes off to do a chore. These little farm children are their parents and ancestors in miniature.

Their young mother, Barbie, comes from the house. She's fine-boned and wears glasses, blonde hair wisping from a perfectly white *Kapp*. "I love her dress," I say of her daughter. "Did you make it?"

She smiles sweetly despite seeming tired. "Yes, I did, thank you. It wasn't hard."

We talk a little about sewing — not that I can, but my mother and sisters do. My son takes sewing lessons too, but I don't mention that, in case it's too modern for her comfort. Traditional gender boundaries are strong here. Barbie's Kapp signals her role as a modest woman and husband's helpmeet.

"I'd sure love to try your milk," I say, peering into the cooler.

"You want to? I'll get you some," says Samuel.

The small cup of milk is fresh and sweet, still warm from the teat. They all watch me. "Do your kids like it?"

"I don't know, they haven't had it," says Samuel.

"No? How about you?"

"None of us drink it," he says, and I realize they see it as a costly commodity.

"Do you have any autism in your community?" I expect not, because it's rumored to be rare among the Amish. No one knows why, but they have a limited gene pool, make their own furniture and clothing, farm traditionally, and encounter less traffic, power sources, and industrial pollution. They consume little alcohol and avoid some medications and medical procedures. All these practices may minimize risk and epigenetic change (a change to the molecules that bind to DNA and alter genetic expression). Still they're not health purists: they eat meat, white flour, and plenty of sugar and buy some plastics and household items.

"I have a relative. That's what they think she has," says Barbie.

"How old is she?"

"In her thirties, I think."

"Does she get any services from the county?"

"I don't know. She stays at home with her family. She seems happy. She's doing some writing and spelling out words lately." She describes it as some kind of typing on a keyboard. "Seems like she likes it," she says, smiling.

"Has she had any camel milk?"

"No."

"Maybe she should try it, since it worked for my son."

"Yes, that's a good idea," she says. Clearly this is a new thought. "We should put our shares together and give her some," she says to the men. They nod, and I see it won't be one person's gesture but a group decision.

"But do you know of any kids, in your group or others, with autism? Or kids that can't talk? Or have really high energy and can't settle down or learn?" Given the size of Amish families (which average seven children per woman), they have quite a few to consider.

"No," say Samuel, Ben, and Barbie thoughtfully. "Can't think of any."

The sun drops lower as my visit nears its end. Ben lives two miles away, a ten-minute trot by buggy, but a neighbor with a car is waiting to give him a lift. "Come visit again or call anytime," he says in that formal cadence.

Samuel and Barbie are leaving for a "wrap-up party." Around fifty Amish families have hosted a food event for the non-Amish community, and money earned from "English" attendees will be "settled" (distributed) among the sponsoring families. Leftover proceeds will fund a local retreat for Amish families to learn about mental illness. Doctors are involved in offering treatment, but Ben later explains to me, "Each family should make its own choice. So often it goes medical when it would not need to. This event is moving toward holistic practices that got lost over the years."

The little girl clambers up on a box, still holding the cat. Her smile is like a sunflower in the barn's late shadows. She'll be a plain-dressed beauty with a largely structured life. It's likely she'll join the church, and a husband, manual labor, and several children will take up her time.

For now she plays in the good dirt and sun, an heirloom seed of this patriarchal life.

Rolling down the driveway, I take a last look. The clothes drying on the line, faded white house paint, scattered farm equipment, and few planted bushes make the place look like my family's farm, though more prosperous in a modest way. And the pleasantly taciturn people aren't that different from my kin.

Things the Amish may not approve of, I did. Uncensored reading, questioning authority, entering competitions, riding motorcycles alone. Wearing pants instead of skirts, getting a high school and college education. But the path that took me from the farm of my childhood led me here. I hold no misty-eyed views of the Amish. I'm too justice-seeking for their *Ordnung*. I'd be pestering the bishops, running a library or women's shelter. But I recognize the value of their ways.

I see the Amish as American pastoralists. They're expanding in number, buying cheaper land in the Midwest, building their networks of stores and workshops. They hire webmasters, use phones, build factories, and meet visitors. Still faith-bound and conservative, they will change when it suits them. After all, they've welcomed camels, such foreigners to their pastures. By the sweat of their brows, they eat bread and tend camels. Their land of milk and honey has gained a new wellspring.

Back home in California, I recall the peaceful feeling of our visit. I call to see how they've been, and Ben answers. "How is John?" I ask.

"He's doing well."

We talk about our kids and our hopes for their futures. And I ask a question that has stayed on my mind. "As a dad, do you ever worry if he'll have trouble finding a mate?"

His answer illuminates his Amish beliefs. "No, not really. Worry begins where faith ends. It will happen if the good Lord's plan is so."

17 A CAMEL MILK SAVIOR

> "Oh! It tastes like milk!"
> — FESTIVAL GOERS

I love our new little camel-milk world. It's cozy and trusting, and everyone is rejoicing. Cameleers from all sorts of places have become my friends online. Thanks to camel milk, Gil and Nancy are finding their camels even more amazing, and Amish farmers are deriving satisfaction from helping others, in their understated way. Kids with autism are talking, rashes are healing, kids and parents are sleeping well. Things are great.

A fifty-year-old friend of mine has severe juvenile-onset rheumatoid arthritis that's limiting his activity. He tries camel milk, drinks eight ounces instead of the four I advised, and becomes so energized that he stays up all night. "I cleaned my *blinds*," he tells me. "I never do that!" He feels so good that he returns to his gym and is also getting more real estate work done. He now drinks four ounces every other day and tells his story to everyone.

Everyone is doing well. Noah sells his milk to customers on trust, receiving payment by check or cash left in his rural mailbox. Marlin shows milking videos online and at lectures. Dallas in Indiana returns calls on Fridays, in the one hour his Amish rules allow him to use the phone. Sam is buying more camels for his herd and dreams of making ice cream. Clyde drops out to pursue other business plans.

I get a Facebook message from someone introducing himself as Walid Abdul-Wahab, from Saudi Arabia. He's a college senior doing a business class project on camel milk, and he wants to visit me. We agree to meet at a local restaurant on Saturday night. When I get there with Tony, I see a pale young man in Western clothes with a scruffy, reddish under-the-chin beard and bright amber eyes.

Walid has been bitten by the camel milk bug and is vibrating with enthusiasm. He's been reselling Amish milk to local Muslims and wants to start a business.

He peppers me with questions. "Do you think you can sell it in the US, and for how much?"

"I could sell it like crazy right now, but I don't want legal challenges. It's illegal to sell raw milk across state lines for human consumption."

"But it is legal to sell camel milk in the US."

"Yes, but raw milk of any kind can be sold in some states, not all."

"What would it take to start a camel milk business in the US?" he asks.

"Raw or pasteurized?"

"Either one."

"People in my community mostly want it raw, with the camels on organic feed, in chemical-free bottles. For a farm you need agriculturally zoned land, some equipment, workers, and camels. Pasteurizing adds more equipment."

"Can you say pasteurized milk has health benefits too?"

"Some people see them, but not many. It's heated for thirty minutes, so that might destroy the enzymes and whatever therapeutic things are in it. There's a market for pasteurized camel milk as a dairy alternative, but it's very small for now."

"But will people drink camel milk? I know Muslims will pay, price is not a big object for them."

"Right now, only desperate people are drinking it," I say. "They're nervous. The number one question is, what does camel milk taste like? Everyone asks that."

"Why, are they afraid their children won't drink it?" asks Walid.

"It's more than that. A camel is no big deal in your part of the world, but here it's odd. There are three kinds of people: the ones who don't want to hear about camel milk; the people who say they should look into it and don't; and the people who say, 'Where do I get it?' and buy it right away."

"Yes, that's true," says Walid sadly. "My price is twenty-four dollars a bottle, because for Muslims, it's a prestigious item, like wine is here. In your home, it is good to offer the guest something special. Like for Ramadan is coming up."

As we chat, I discover he doesn't realize the difference between state law and FDA regulations. But he seems uninterested.

Tony asks, "If you've been doing this for a year, why did you only contact Christina now?"

"You were the first person I was told about," he says, looking at me. "But I didn't know anything. I didn't have anything to offer you yet." He almost blushes. It's kind of sweet.

We talk about his family, who own a steel company back home. His mother is half-Syrian. She does not veil her face, although Walid wants her to: she only wears an abaya with her hair showing. His city of Jeddah is quite modern, he says, and many women don't wear the veil, but he believes they should. In his view, "The veil is worn by people who wish to say, 'I am dedicated to exploring and getting closer to God, so back off from me.'" He says he avoids alcohol, doesn't date, works out, and worships regularly. He has Arabic script and a large camel sticker on his milk-white SUV.

Then he asks, "What do you think about Marlin?"

"Marlin is great. He's convinced the Constitution protects him." I explain how just being accused of causing sickness in a person can get you slammed by a lawsuit. I suggest Walid get liability insurance. But he's hoping for an easier way.

"I know this Lebanese Republican congressman. He says with enough money and the right people, making raw milk legal to ship across state lines can be done."

"That's true," I tell him. "I just never had money to pay those people. A lobbyist and big donations would do it." We sigh and drink our tea.

"Do you drink camel milk every day?" I ask.

"Only when I order it. Do you?"

"Yes, we all drink it," says Tony.

"At home, I just tell my driver to go find a Bedouin by the side of the road, and they milk it, and that's it."

As I try again to explain legal and liability issues to Walid, it's clear he doesn't know what I mean. And it seems he just doesn't care. I ask if he's a US citizen. He isn't.

"So at worst, you can be deported or something," I say. "Fly away home, and you just can't come back."

"Or come back later when it's done," he says.

"Do you have someone to pay your legal bills, if you sell raw milk and get in trouble?"

"Oh, no. I have a sort of diplomatic relationship."

"So you are immune, really."

"Yes, I can just leave, and it will be okay. I can come back when it's all over. I don't think they can do anything to me."

Then I get it. He is basically able to manipulate, buck, and maybe even finance the entire system. He might be a camel milk savior.

"You might be the perfect person to do this!" I exclaim. I don't really like his lack of legal responsibility, but no American big-money types have invested in what they think is a small niche product. So I guess if he's going to do it, I'll help him do it right.

Walid soon invites me to an Islamic food festival near my home where he plans to sell camel milk. As far as we know, it's the first time it will be sold in public in the United States. In a grassy park by a table labeled "America's first and finest camel milk," he's pitching forty pints of fresh Amish milk as a special Ramadan treat.

"The big bottle is fifty dollars, and here's an eight-ounce bottle for sixteen dollars," he says.

"Hardly anyone's here," I say, worried for him.

"My people like to come later, not early." But friends and a cousin are here to support him, all clean-cut, fit young men. "Hey, tell her about your dad's camels," Walid says to one.

Yasir smiles shyly. He has hazel eyes behind glasses that match his sandy-blond hair. Like Walid, he doesn't look stereotypically Saudi. Already I'm learning some things I didn't know.

"My dad has a ranch," he says. "He likes to go to the camels on weekend mornings. Feed them, spend time with them."

"Does he drink the milk?"

"He does, but not raw. He says it upsets his stomach that way."

"So he heats it?"

"Yes, when he wants a little."

"People from Saudi think the milk gives them diarrhea," says Walid.

"I hear just the opposite from users in Israel and the US, who treat their Crohn's and irritable bowel syndrome with it, so that's puzzling," I say.

We watch people walk by, hesitate, and leave.

"Hey, we're visiting the Millers' Amish farm again," says Tony. Walid's never been there. "With your beard, just put on a straw hat and black clothes, and you'll blend right in. They'll think you're Amish," Tony teases.

"Or blow-dry your hair and trim it around your face in a bowl cut," I joke.

"I don't know if they would think I was one of them or not," he says seriously.

It's funny and ironic to think of these rule-bound religions colliding, when both originated from small rural communities, have strict behavior customs, and mandate beards for men and head and body coverings for women. With that much in common, Walid and Amos should start a farm together.

A knot of onlookers grows.

"Camel milk?" they say.

"What do you do with it?"

"You can drink it?"

And the familiar question: "What does it taste like?"

Walid offers samples in little paper cups. People stare at them and sip, shivering with fear. "Oh! It tastes like milk!" they say. Relief, wonderment, and smiles abound.

Walid sells no milk for the next two hours. Ramadan sales are a bust.

He returns two weeks later to borrow some milk from me for a school business competition. "I was on a conference call with a very rich Middle Eastern guy and my friend. I was talking about camel milk. The rich guy says, 'Camel milk? That gives me diarrhea!'"

Do Arab people have more sensitive guts, or is the milk somehow different? I research the issue and learn it's probably not the milk — it's more likely to be caused by bacterial contamination in handling or storage. After all, their society was once fueled by it.

But we don't have to drink milk from camels stopped by the roadside. Even without electricity, the Amish employ modern, hygienic methods of handling raw and pasteurized milk. Perhaps they have something to share with the Bedouins and other nomads. Modern wisdom might be springing from some old and surprising sources.

18 A FUNDAMENTAL EVOLUTION

"This evolution stuff is really crazy."
— MARLIN TROYER

At the next Oasis Camel Clinic at Gil and Nancy's, Walid comes to meet the American camel world. Marlin is there with his wife, Savannah, in her modest dress and white head covering. After Marlin teaches us how to milk, using a pink plastic udder attached to the picnic table, he and Walid start talking by the dinner buffet. Two muscular young men with wagging under-chin beards, they are mirror images from different worlds.

Marlin grew up as one of eleven kids on various farms, with harsh weather flapping their plastic-taped windows. He remembers scooping warm cow manure to treat a cut foot. Like most Amish boys, he left school after eighth grade. Once he was old enough, he started a wood furniture company, then sold it. His success has enabled him to indulge his longing for exotic animals. He married a woman who covers her head.

Walid was born abroad, attended international schools, is graduating from the University of Southern California (locally nicknamed the University of Spoiled Children), and lives in a luxury apartment in downtown Los Angeles. His family's wealth enables him to start a quixotic camel-milk company. He plans to marry a woman who veils her face and head.

I can see their connection growing, folded arms angling toward each other as their bodies draw closer.

"This evolution stuff is really crazy," Marlin says.

"Yes, I know," Walid says.

"It doesn't make sense. If you look at the science, creationism has the answers."

"It really does," Walid agrees.

After the clinic, they begin communicating. Walid decides to abandon the Muslim market and target the parents of kids with autism, so he calls me all the time for advice. Soon he's out visiting Noah in Pennsylvania and other farmers, hoping to resell their milk. He tried to offer some of them Qur'ans to read, but they countered with their Bibles and declined. He's also offering them seven dollars per sixteen-ounce bottle, enough for some, but Marlin, who's wildly independent, says no.

Now Walid is ready to set up his website, and I work with him for very little, writing and editing the copy, keeping his science references clean, and deleting false or far-fetched claims that might provoke the FDA. He says he'll pay the rest of my fee once he's made money. But I just want him to succeed. I help most of the farmers with their websites, labels, and marketing copy (mostly in exchange for milk, or for a token fee just to remind them that women's labor should be compensated). And so far everyone's getting along fine.

I get a shock when I see a picture of an angelic-looking Amish man on Walid's website. I wonder how he did that, since Amish don't like to be photographed. Then I look past the suspenders and hat and recognize Walid's face. "What?" I say aloud to myself. "How is this even allowed?" I gently ask Walid if he'd carefully considered the consequences, but he's proud and doesn't see a problem. I expect the photos to anger Marlin, but he just shrugs it off. "Lots of people use Amish imagery to make money, he's just another one."

Then Marlin starts to worry. He thinks Walid will drive the farmers' prices down. "I heard he wants to get to five dollars a bottle. That's total starvation wages!"

I hope he's wrong. But to me Walid confirms his goal of getting his cost down to six or maybe even five dollars a bottle. "That's to create greater returns for the investor and interest a major beverage company, like Coca-Cola," he says.

When farmers can sell camel milk for nine to twelve dollars per bottle from their own farms, why would they sell for half price to Walid? They are pastoralists, focused on animals and land, not much different from Negev Bedouins or the Tuareg in Niger. Marlin and Noah don't sell to stores. And their use of phones and email is restricted. Most nomads and pastoralists aren't into writing, lobbying lawmakers, or making flashy websites.

I wish I could help them sell milk online, especially raw. A hygienic raw-milk operation is exceedingly low risk, and no one in the United States has reported getting sick. But like Gil and Nancy, I don't want to get sued. Marlin and the Amish have their community as a backup if they did. Walid can flee the country without consequences. But I can't handle more stress. So I remain the fundamentalists' adviser, researcher, and patient listener, just helping them get the milk to the kids who need it.

Walid calls. "What did you call that insurance? A liability policy? I need to buy one."

Then he says, "A California grocery chain just ordered twelve frozen bottles."

"Camel milk finally in a store — in the open! That's amazing," I say.

I think of my suitcases of camel milk rolling through LAX, San Diego, Atlanta, and JFK, holding thousand-dollar Styrofoam cases sprinkled with brown Bedouin dust. No more doctor's letters, ice-packed coolers, or pricey airline tickets are needed. Now parents can go to the store, pick up a bottle, and give it to their child that day. If Walid's scheme works, the miracle can keep growing. It's good news for camels and the farmers who care for them as well as for the kids.

One Friday, I volunteer to work at Walid's booth at a food trade show, so he can take time out to pray. While he's gone, I spot a Whole Foods executive. I give him a tiny cup of milk and explain the special properties. I get his business card and give it to Walid, who's very happy. They arrange a call. Bottles appear in Whole Foods markets! It's a crowning achievement. (It costs twenty-six dollars a bottle.)

I speak to more doctors and lecture at conferences. And I finally meet Dr. Amnon Gonenne, who visits my town. Thoughtful and courteous, he's everything I expected. Our early exchanges have flowered into a movement.

Soon a public health expert asks me to write a case report for a peer-reviewed medical journal. It describes my son's background and his experience with camel milk. Titled "Autism Spectrum Disorder Treated with Camel Milk," it appears in print and online. It is the article I once hoped to find.

When I go on a TV show to talk about the article, some scientists hear the news. The report will take me across the world to spread the word about camels.

19 YOU KNOWS NOTHING ABOUT CAMEL

"Tell me about yourself."
— CAMELEER INDIA

As word about camel milk spreads, and my articles and videos are seen online, my Facebook page becomes a hive of camel activity. People start writing to me, not just parents but camel people. I'd like to know more about the international camel scene, but I keep things buttoned up online and rarely read junk messages ("Hi, pretty lady, where do you live, call me," the usual). But I let some new messages in. I never knew this many men wanted to talk about camels. Fuzzy photos arrive from rural villages in faraway countries. Many feature thin, dark-haired guys in sandals, with camels. One of the men goes by the screen name of Cameleer India.

> Hi. Hello. How are you Hey I am fine.
> Whats the camel milk news from you?
> Do you like to drink camel milk
> Hello.
> What are you doing
> Wats up dear
> Somebody is there

I don't answer his messages because I'm not sure what this is. Is he serious, a flirt, or just bored? Two days later, he posts some strange and interesting animal and camel pictures on my personal page. I like the iridescent black chickens and lumbering water buffalo, but some pictures show thin, mangy dogs. Because of some weird glitch, I can't remove them, so I decide to message him back.

ME: Hi there...I hope you are fine. Can you take the photos off
   my page? I don't have room for that many pictures...thank
   you!
CAMELEER: Ok
   I will if you don't like them
   You should visit Bikaner once

Bikaner? Home to the main camel research center of India? Now I'm interested. Located near the border with Pakistan, it's home to many camels. But the center's website is hard to navigate, and no one returns my emails. If Cameleer is offering me a chance to learn about it, why not?

CAMELEER: I am studying post graduation at Bikaner research
   center, specializing in livestock production and management
ME: Excellent!
CAMELEER: There a lot of products are prepared from camel milk
ME: What kind of products from camels?
CAMELEER: Milk products like coffee, some sweets like gulab
   jamun, peda, rasgulla, ice cream, lassi and milk powder is
   made there
ME: Yummy
CAMELEER: Ya it is
CAMELEER: How old are you
ME: I'm older than you probably...I have a teenage son.
CAMELEER: Ok Whats your hobbies
ME: I've gotta go to a meeting now...have a great week!
CAMELEER: Ok good night

It seems like this fellow is young and not yet established. He's probably not a scientist who can arrange a university visit. He strikes me as a livestock helper, although I don't know for sure. I won't be going to Bikaner to work with him. But I'd like to learn about Indian camels.

The next day, he sends photos of himself holding a plate of chana masala (spiced chickpeas), a wistful look in his eyes. I say, "That looks nice, I had it in India." He says to come back and he'll make it for me. I say I've been to Haryana. We talk more about animals, and I think it's productive.

Days later, I must contact him again. The latest picture he's posted on my page is one of some kind of animal fornicating. While it's quirky and interesting, I suspect it may set a bad precedent. Allowing sex talk of any kind is risky with men, even if it only concerns livestock.

ME: Hey Cameleer, can you take this one down please? Thank
    you —
CAMELEER: ok dear
    hello
    Hello
    R u busy

He's too intense with the messaging, so I ignore him. But he's back every day for a week:

CAMELEER: Hi
    Wanna to come to Haryana
    Where are you busy
    Hello
    What are you doing
    Hi how are you

Finally I message him. He's now posting dozens of pictures on my Facebook page. To make it worse, I still can't remove them. They are pretty cool, like a blurry *National Geographic* spread, with skinny camels, wild birds with wings splayed, and a mélange of dogs, buffalo, and livestock we'd consider exotic in the United States. It's like a free trip to Bikaner! But they take up far too much space. He says he is sorry.

Three days later:

ME: Hi…this is my last request…PLEASE take your photos off my Facebook page…they keep appearing and i want them OFF.

CAMELEER: Ok I forgot that

ME: Thank u

CAMELEER: what are you doing now

ME: Writing a new magazine article on camels. I'll post it in two months when it comes out.

CAMELEER: ok wanna came to Haryana again
yesterday I prepare a cheese recipe

He sends a picture of himself holding a steamy dish of paneer, the Indian cheese, beside a stove in his small kitchen.

However intermittently annoying and interesting Cameleer is, he's not as bad as the faraway businessman who asks for a video meeting, then mostly talks about how I look like his favorite actress. Most men who write me from other countries are autism dads, always respectful and sweet. But their animal experience is limited to buying sheep to sacrifice for the poor at religious festivals. They don't own camels and can't offer any scientific lore.

Next day:

CAMELEER: hi today i posted a video have u seen it

It is a fascinating video of Indian men helping camels mate. They lift up the male's body and help him climb onto the female's back to penetrate her. This is real "animal husbandry," as they are helping the "husband" camel. I don't get why one man is thwacking the male camel's tail very hard with a stick while the camel's literally trying to get his hump on.

ME: Why is the man hitting him?
CAMELEER: he rub the hump with stick and give gentle strock of
    stick to excite him
    you should visit bikaner and pushkar fair the biggest camel
    market of world
    if you have not seen these you knows nothing about camel
    tell me about yourself
    Go take some photos for me in there and send them!
ME: I am married so i am busy with my family.

Married means the same in any culture. I try to be polite after this, but his messages keep coming. Finally, I totally ignore him.

Two days later:

CAMELEER: hello... what are you doing

Two weeks later:

CAMELEER: Hiiiiiiiiiiiiiiiiiiiiiiiii

This repeats several times, until I block him.

Months later, a Facebook cameleer posts that a guy sent her pictures of reproductive organs — his own. Another woman says, "Me too." It was Cameleer India.

Oh Cameleer, I'll miss the animals in your life. I will never eat your cheese dish or come to Haryana. True, you know more about camels than I do, but I know way too much about you.

20 CAMEL FARM HEAVEN

"Yasalaam, how wonderful and fantastic!"

— CAMEL RACE ANNOUNCER

The email asking if I'll come to Dubai feels like a hot desert wind. The idea of visiting the large camel farm there has long shimmered like a mirage in my mind. I've heard they have thousands of camels and are trying to export milk to the United States.

The next email is from Dr. Jutka Juhász, the farm's chief veterinarian. She saw my case report and says she wants to meet, to learn about autism and help make camel milk accessible to people who need it. They've named their milk Camelicious. According to Kirsten, the company's PR representative, "Supporting the traditions of Dubai and the United Arab Emirates is important to the sheikh and camels are an expression of that tradition." After all, this is a culture that once depended on camels. Some influential people display favorite dead camels, stuffed, in their homes.

While autism consumers often prefer raw milk, Camelicious is pasteurized, but it's flash-pasteurized, heated only for seconds. Some feel this helps preserve the milk's properties better than traditional pasteurization methods do. On a video call, Kirsten says that the Central Veterinary Research Lab in Dubai, founded by the sheikh, "did a little trial with ten autistic kids and eight responded very notably to camel milk." This is a path worth exploring.

"Will you do some speaking?" she asks.

"Sure. What should I know about cultural sensitivities? You know my milk came from Israel."

"We call it Palestine."

"And my milk came from Bedouins."

"And Bedouins are usually Muslim," she replies.

"Right…so I should say my milk came from Bedouins in Palestine? But what part of Israel is Palestine?"

She shrugs. "You can call all of it Palestine. That's what they call it."

"So can I say it came from Bedouins in the Middle East?"

"No, because then they will ask what country, and when you went there."

"I've never been there."

"So it's Palestine and you've never been there."

I don't want to set off cultural land mines. I just want to help people. I am neutral, the Switzerland of camel milk.

Camelicious has just launched their products in London, with camel cappuccinos and a guy in a camel costume running a charity race. I hope they will launch in the United States next, but the US government keeps stalling the approval process.

Camelicious comes under the aegis of Sheikh Mohammed bin Rashid Al Maktoum, vice president and prime minister of the United Arab Emirates and ruler of the Emirate of Dubai. My contacts who know him say, "Sheikh is very smart. He manages things brilliantly. He oversees many challenges in his country and does it all well." And helping to transform Dubai from a remote, pearl-diving village into its current incarnation as a modern, high-rise city and global business center is a staggering achievement, even given the boost from trade and investment money and low-cost imported labor.

Standing in the departure line for my Emirates Airline flight is like being in a foreign country already. I'm the only blonde in sight: other women passengers display shiny black hair or headscarves and long dresses. Emirates flight attendants, all young, wear a red-trimmed tan suit, and the uniform hat has an attached white veil that drapes becomingly down the chest. It's an allusion to veiled women, yet it beckons observers to admire their faces. They wear the required full makeup, red lips, and coiffed hairstyles, mostly chignons or buns, and even the few men are handsome. So begins my next immersion into this older, more gender-defined world.

After the sixteen-hour nonstop flight from Los Angeles, emerging into Dubai Airport is like entering the outer halls of heaven. The customs officers wear long white robes, ceilings are the height of European cathedrals, and impossibly tall chrome columns and silver Rolex wall clocks dazzle a traveler's weary eyes. Tony is with me; we rise silently in clear glass elevators past tiles trickling with water, afloat in a contemporary void. Lights glow far above. Emirates passport control is largely silent, staffed by somber men and women, their heads covered. A large camel statue stands near the gift shops. I look for the machine dispensing twenty-four-karat-gold bars that's said to be a feature of the airport, but I can't find it. Maybe that's in the VIP section.

Kirsten, the PR agent, picks us up. She's friendly, kindly ignoring the fact that my black clothes are covered with white lint from the airline blanket. We settle into her gray sedan, unusual only for the fire extinguisher strapped to the front seat floor.

"So why do you have a fire extinguisher?"

"The emergency services aren't the best sometimes, so you never know."

Down Sheikh Zayed Road, the main route into Dubai City, monolithic buildings have risen even more fantastically in the five years since I first saw them, creating a skyline of sinuous shapes and tall rectangles. The Rotana Hotel has a perfumed lobby with exotic flower arrangements, curved arches, and navy and purple fabrics.

In the morning, Kirsten drives us along curving modern roads, lined with flowers and new skyscrapers, to Umm Nahad, where the farm lies in a wide expanse of flat sand. The two-lane highway is almost camouflaged in the empty desert, the gray-white landscape tinged with brown and scattered with rocks. Single hillocks of grass and a few trees dot the roadside. A royal residence is out this way, and a military jet roars from a nearby air force base. Eventually, we see a stand of mature green trees marking the perimeter of the farm.

As the car turns up the lane, I see purple and gold buildings bearing the scripted letters "EICMP" (standing for Emirates Industries for Camel Milk Products) shining in the morning sun. We stop at the entry gates, are waved cheerily through, and roll into a sunny park populated by birds.

We pass purple trucks decorated with white waves of milk, then park by a building in back. I'm nervous, because to me this land of camel milk is special ground. I am introduced to Dr. Jutka, as everyone calls her, a tall, brown-eyed Hungarian woman with short, wavy black hair. She welcomes Tony and me in her slightly accented English and says to call her Jutka. We then meet the management. I'm unsure whether businessmen in this conservative Muslim country will want to shake hands with me, but they extend theirs with courtesy, and we engage in small talk. Then Jutka, Tony, Kirsten, and I settle in the conference room under gold-framed portraits of three of the United Arab Emirates royals in regal white head coverings.

Small bottles of pasteurized camel milk are brought in on a tray, adorned with different colorful cartoon camels to match their flavors: chocolate, strawberry, date, and saffron. The bottle of plain milk is purple and white, with no cartoon. "Emirates CAMEL Goodness," the label reads. This polished packaging is a long way from the handwritten bottle tops of the Amish.

I sip the plain milk, and my mouth puckers a little after I taste the initial sweetness; the pasteurization enhances the presence of salt. The date milk, flavored with date syrup, is delicious. The thinner, slightly sweet saffron flavor is aimed at the Asian market. The chocolate milk, made with cocoa powder, tastes like normal US chocolate milk, but without the usual thick aftertaste.

"Would you like to see the camels?" I always want to see camels, and nowhere else am I likely to see this many. So we pull blue booties over our shoes to prevent the farm from being contaminated by hitchhiking germs, and step out into the sun. In Jutka's SUV we pass through the main campus and enter a stunning landscape of ocher sand. A mirage seems to waver through the warm air. It turns out to be a field of reddish-copper camels with coats glimmering like silk.

My mouth falls open.

"How many are there?"

"Probably around 3,700 now. We plan to get to 5,000 at least."

They gleam and glow, these unearthly camels, standing or gently milling about, with waving manes and dune-like humps.

"How do you get them to shine like that?"

"They are washed once a month," she says.

More and more camels flash by, untethered and content: blond, sandy, brown, gold, all the colors of a desert dream. They are separated by gender and function. Here are the yearling males, kicking their feet up together. Here are a few bulls, seemingly tall and taciturn when not in rut. Here are around three hundred milking moms, kept with their babies for a year, until around the time they naturally stop nursing. Recently weaned babies are kept in pastures adjacent to their mothers for a month, so they don't feel separated. We pass one group of babies currently being weaned, who honk and groan, causing a ripple reaction in another group. "'Oh, I'm missing my mommy.' 'I'm missing mine too,'" Jutka translates, a mother herself.

On and on we go, through fields as organized as a painting. There's even a large walking track for the camels' leisure. Compared to their nomadic brethren, these camels live pampered lives.

In the conference room, we eat a lunch of fish curry and lamb and rice biryani, and I adopt their custom of using tissues for napkins. The farm manager, Dr. Peter Nagy, also a vet, comes in, and we get his viewpoints too.

After lunch, we go to the white-tiled camel surgery and treatment suite. The size of an American firehouse, it has three tall blue stalls, as camels are more comfortable standing rather than lying during most medical procedures. Here baby camels are conceived through artificial insemination, ailments are treated, and scientific boundaries are pushed. Jutka pulls out a triangular probe with a small cord attached. It's an ultrasound device that can verify pregnancy as early as thirteen days after conception, a great advantage over the traditional guesswork of watching for uncertain pregnancy signs like the tail "flag" and self-isolation. "It goes in the rectum," she says. "Many animals won't tolerate it, but the camels are fine. I can use it for all kinds of things, to check what's going on." To do surgery, "we just put something down, and the camel lies on the floor."

This airy, cool building also holds a lab where camel sperm is used to fertilize eggs in a petri dish. Jutka returns from the lab, slips on a long green plastic glove, squirts it with gel and reaches elbow-deep into the female's vaginal canal to implant some embryos. No wonder she has such admirable arm muscles. (That and yoga.)

During a quick break, I sample the raw camel milk. Our hosts are eager for my reaction, since I've tasted camel milk from so many sources. I tip the tiny paper cup into my mouth, and it's the most palatable, smooth-tasting milk I've ever had. "No antibiotics, very natural," Jutka says.

"Yes, I can taste it," I say. There's no flavor of grass, well water, grain, or any of the slight hints that give raw camel milks their own signature, like fine cheeses. These camels eat hay, vitamins, and minerals (and maybe some bran), but here in the desert, they don't get fresh grass.

We head outdoors, passing through what resembles a desert meditation garden, to observe the afternoon milking. Birds trill and call "whoo-whoo" as they flutter through the sparse trees. Now I'll observe camels doing what they may not do anywhere else (except at the hands of Gil and maybe some nomads) — give milk without their babies initiating the flow. From a viewing platform above the modern outdoor milking area, we watch as a signal is given and the camels drift into the shining stalls in a slow, regal line. A couple of workmen attach milking machines to their udders. Their precious milk flows through a network of tubes to a separate refrigerated processing facility. No human hands touch it. The system, designed and installed by a specialized British milking-parlor provider, tracks each camel's output from the twice-daily milking of five to six liters a day. (The 5 a.m. milking accounts for roughly 70 percent of production, and the 3 p.m. milking for the rest.) If a problem is detected with a given camel, the system won't allow it to be milked.

So calm and efficient is the scene, it's like these majestic mothers milk themselves. "Good breeding" has increased milk production, and Jutka is aiming for twenty liters per head. (The farm does not use artificial hormones, she says.) "Good training" is why the camels give their milk so freely — although camels won't give milk if they're not happy, so apparently they are satisfied as well.

We wind up our day with a visit to "the gang," a gossipy lineup of retired camels, from twenty-five to thirty-five years old, standing behind a low concrete wall. Caramel, tan, beige, and mocha, their mouths purse and their brown eyes shine with interest under long, curling lashes. I insert whole carrots like thermometers into their mouths, and they munch with jaws sliding sideways, their lower lips drooping with satisfaction. A dozen camels thrust their flirty faces forward, and I laugh. "They know the drill, don't they?" I ask Jutka.

"Yes, greeting people is their job now, and they are good at it!" she says, beaming fondly at them.

I turn to see two dozen men in tan coveralls, matching caps, and black boots. They are some of the Camelicious workers. Jutka has worked mightily to assist them, as they are largely from other countries. She says they get housing, assistance with health problems, and gentle support for workforce grooming and hygiene.

That night we return to the Rotana Hotel, but no trip is complete without going to the Dubai Mall. It's not just huge, it's colossal. The old must-do mall had a ski slope, but this one holds a massive aquarium, enormous sculptures, and dancing fountains that rival Las Vegas. European tourists mingle with Arab women in full-length black, some with *niqab*s, and men in head-to-toe white robes and thick leather sandals. (Often tourists want to photograph their traditional attire, but it's against the law without their consent.) In a gilded hideaway evoking a classic *souk* (market), I spot crystal-trimmed women's robes, rare wool scarves, and heavy gold floral tea sets. I walk through a keyhole-shaped arch and stop short at the sight of an enormous falcon sitting on its handler's arm. Like the camel, it's a symbol of Arab desert culture. "Come, touch, it's okay," the handler says.

"Touch the bird?"

"Yes, it's fine, you will see."

I look at the bird's eye, anchored in its own remote reality. I stroke its head with a finger. It feels softer than down or silk. I look into the circle of its eye and see infinite depths, speaking of mountains and rocks and sun. I shiver at the bird's intelligence, a type far different from my own. This bird may be tethered inside a mall, but its essence is not bound to this earth.

Next day we head to the pristine new Majlis Café, an EICMP-associated project serving gourmet camel-milk products. It's located in the meeting place ("majlis") adjacent to the imposing Jumeirah mosque. Today I will speak to parents, professionals, and journalists about camel milk, autism, and other issues. My talk is the first public event ever held here, they tell me. The café has a beige marble floor and a double staircase of dark golden-tipped wood. White sofas left-over from a royal wedding are arranged before a gleaming bar offering camel milk lattes, hot chocolate, ice cream, and small, jewel-colored muffins. White friezes in the Islamic style accent the creamy walls.

Men in suits and women in smart daytime wear, a few wearing headscarves, start to arrive. I ask where they come from. Many are well-to-do expatriates; some are journalists. I meet Dr. Hibah Shata, a Saudi doctor, proud mother of a child with autism, and the founder of the Child Early Intervention Medical Center. She will host the Autism Awareness Gala later this week. Powerful and stylish in her dark suit and floral blouse, she's a wholehearted supporter of helping the kids. Jutka and Kirsten are here as well.

"I am happy to be here, in a country with a long history of camel milk, in this week of Autism Awareness," I say. I describe my son's and other children's positive experiences with camel milk: better language and attention, increased sleep and emotional expressions, hugging people, needed weight gain, and improvement in skin conditions. I explain possible causes of these effects. When I invite the audience to contribute, a mother in a black robe and teal headscarf points at three bright-eyed, black-haired young children eating ice cream.

"My son has autism and it helped him improve, and my youngest child, who has a cow milk allergy, can finally drink milk," she says. She has toted along the tallest bottle of camel milk I've ever seen. She delivers an intense impromptu mini-lecture on special diets, then others ask questions, and I give some interviews to journalists.

It's lunchtime, and the chefs are eager to offer special dishes featuring camel milk. I sink onto a white banquette and nibble a leaf-green muffin. It's pistachio, and so good, without a hint of camel flavor. They bring me some vanilla ice cream and a plate holding four neatly trimmed tea sandwiches. I eat one, and it's delicious. "What is this?" I ask the smiling young chef.

"Ma'am, the inside is mortadella. Made from yearlings, so it's very good."

Oh, it's camel meat. It's similar to Italian prosciutto but less salty, milder, and more tender. "This is really good," I say to Jutka. "Did you try it?"

She smiles slightly. "No, thanks," she says, and turns away.

I realize suddenly that these are her babies — the young males that have no practical use on a milk farm. I see what looks like a film of tears in her eyes and feel slightly horrified. I finish eating a second sandwich, unwilling to waste this precious meat, but I'm embarrassed to be consuming her loved ones. After a few minutes, I say, "I'm sorry, I didn't know." She kindly assures me not to worry, but I can see her pain's better left alone.

Next day we're on the cover of the *Khaleej Times*, and inside is a full-page section with photos of me and the mother of three with her son. She holds him in an anguished pose, and I see the suffering that her tough facade concealed yesterday. Despite the polish, the luxury, the fun, and social chat, we mothers hurt — because our kids hurt, with their various ailments; their rejection from schools, social settings, and sometimes family circles; their inability to speak; their frustrations; their intelligent minds struggling for expression. This is what matters. It's as if camels formed a metaphorical caravan that brought me here to join them.

For the rest of the week, I participate in deep discussions about camels and their milk — biology, ecology, psychology — with Jutka, Tony, Peter, and Kirsten, with others chiming in. There is much to learn and do.

One day Tony, Jutka, and I don white lab coats, blue hairnets, and matching shoe covers and enter the gleaming milk-processing plant. I taste a soft cheese studded with caraway seeds, similar to a very mild feta. "It took four long years to make a good cheese," says Chinnakonda Thulasiram, the Indian plant manager, as they had to experiment with the unique characteristics of camel milk fats, enzymes, and other components. Now the milk is starting to gain a commercial footing, and the cheese goes to fine hotels.

They've also made a yogurt for drinking, called laban, lassi, or kefir in different countries, which he says uses healthy probiotic cultures. But as a true dairy scientist, he's not totally satisfied with its thickness and launches into an explanation of why working with camel milk is so challenging.

"We don't do anything artificial — should be natural, natural, natural. And you need the patience, and sometimes, at the end of the day, you are a human being." He grins below his hairnet.

A low hum fills this echoingly clean factory, where they also make powdered camel milk, inside huge dryers that heat the milk to 325 degrees Fahrenheit. Liquid milk must be sold quickly, "but if we make it a powder, you can sell it for one year," Chinnakonda says. The dried milk meets European Union food standards. "We wanted the best quality powder." He points through the clear glass windows at two installations resembling missile silos. These are freeze dryers, which chill the milk under a vacuum, removing the water and preserving "99.9 percent" of the nutritional value in the remaining solids, he says. But the process is slow and costly.

"It takes whole twenty-four hours, all your refrigeration, heavy pump, electrical — and production is too low. It's just like gold for us." Yet they persevere.

Jutka has goals for her camels that go beyond gourmet products. One of her dreams is to offer camel therapy to autistic kids. Another is conducting a clinical trial to show that camel milk is effective for treating autism. We've planned a collaboration, and I'll help design the trial. She takes me to an autism therapy center in Dubai Healthcare City, one of the centralized, park-like enclaves dedicated to media, healthcare, education, and other purposes. We have a great meeting, and the providers are eager to participate in the trial.

For World Autism Awareness Day, which has a "Light it up blue" theme, I put on a long, strapless blue dress, make it modest with a scarf, and travel to Jumeirah Beach Hotel, a resort near the towering, sail-shaped Burj Al Arab, the world's only seven-star hotel. The closest I got to camels on my last trip here was sipping a camel milk cocktail in the Burj's lavish sky-high bar. So it feels good to be among like-minded people at tonight's autism gala. White- and blue-skirted table-cloths adorn dozens of tables by the Arabian Gulf. As evening falls, a puzzle piece, the symbol representing autism's complexity, appears in glowing blue light on the side of the Burj. When it's my turn, I stand on the brightly lit stage and explain how the camel is helping autism families everywhere. "*Shukran*," I manage to say, an Arabic expression of thanks. Afterward, people crowd around to talk. Two eager young boys ask to pose for pictures with me for a school project on autism. Their hopeful smiles strike at my heart, reminding me how empathetic neurotypical children can be toward those with autism when encouraged. It's not a trait I've seen much before — maybe these kids will help things change.

The next day in Media City, I tape an interview for the show *Studio One* on Dubai One TV. Even the show's hosts are excited about the milk.

With a modern bus and rail system, the city is very easy to get around, and it boasts amusements like cooling off at waterparks (such as the Wild Wadi, which has a women's day), inspecting jaw-dropping buildings, driving racecars, and shopping. It's less easy to access older traditions. I've already tried most of the tourist desert activities: surfing sand dunes (scorching my bare feet in the burning-hot sand), dune bashing (a scream-provoking tumble over sliding hills of sand), sitting on a tethered camel, and drinking tea in a desert tent. But this visit is far better.

A friendly Camelicious executive takes us to see fresh camel legs for sale in a butcher shop, and we eat camel burgers and hot dogs (the burger is great, but the dog is best drowned in ketchup). Tony and I visit the old souks down by Dubai Creek, the site of the early pearl-diving village that gave way to the modern metropolis. Here, as in other areas, huge photos of Sheikh Mohammed and other royals appear on public walls and signs. Five years ago, this area was much more conservative and working class, with male laborers from India and other countries averting their eyes from me in alleys hung with marigolds and scarves. (In Islamic countries, looking deliberately at a woman other than a relative or spouse can be viewed as disrespectful.) Now their faces look happier, and a few don't shy away from my accidental glances. We go deeper into the immigrant quarter, where merchants sell affordable goods from India, Pakistan, and Tibet. Then we walk through Deira, into the arched buildings of the spice market, brimming with baskets of vermilion, orange, and green powders, and pass the gold souk's glittering windows of rich-yellow twenty-two-karat-gold jewelry. I see mannequins in gold-link miniskirts and a suit made entirely of gold mesh.

Our last day is all about camels. We taxi out to a large desert fairground for the Al-Marmoom Heritage Festival, an annual celebration of Emirati traditions. There are thousands of camels, in herds and knots, tethered to poles, standing on hillocks, and cushing by a racetrack. White tents are equipped with lounges, loudspeakers, and satellite dishes. Trainers watch over small groups of camels the color of white stone. These are racing camels, lean as whippets, with loins curved for speed.

The sun shines on several dealerships' worth of new cars, plus rows and rows of identical SUVs that will be offered as prizes.

Jutka picks us up in her own SUV, and we head for the milking competition, held in a parking lot blanketed in red carpets. Tents with more white couches and overstuffed chairs hold Emirati men of all ages in starched white *dishdasha*s, *kandura*s, or *thobe*s. Red-checked scarves called *ghutra*s frame their artfully scruffed faces, held by circled black cords called *agal*s, inspired by Bedouin camel ropes. Two men greet each other among the tea-drinking loungers, pressing their noses and foreheads together with affection.

These camel owners have come from all over for the festival. There are thousands of men, maybe outnumbering the camels. Jutka and I are the only women I've seen. I have a surprising urge to cover my face, but I feel welcome and totally safe. I'm super fair-skinned and burn in a flash, so I drape my scarf to block out the sun. Jutka doesn't even bother with a hat — she just wears jeans and her usual polo shirt.

Now it's contest time. Workers in baggy pants and plaid shirts rapidly milk camels and pour the foaming milk from blue plastic buckets into wide metal bowls to be measured. Prizes are awarded for speed and output. The Camelicious team, in blue polo shirts and khaki hats, wear surgical masks. Jutka moves among them, supervising, and when their winning results are announced, she pauses for a proud smile. "I'm busy now, but someone will take you around," she says to me. "He's a Bedouin, a good friend."

A tall man in a white thobe picks us up in an SUV. Around the vast eight-kilometer racetrack (it expands to ten kilometers), groups of camels, some with halters and some covered with blankets, are tied up awaiting races or prospective buyers. Our driver's English is scant, but we communicate with gestures and expressions. We idle among a large crowd of SUVs by the track, apparently waiting for something. A tea hawker comes by, and I order a cup. Before he can bring it to me, the driver suddenly gestures for me to close my door. Then we're off, driving on the racetrack.

Over the radio comes the voice of the announcer, in the auctioneers' tones of race announcers everywhere, but in Arabic. We are moving in a tight group of white and beige SUVs carrying Emirati and other Arab men. Then I realize we're *in* the race. On the track to our left, small fabric-covered robots are strapped atop the camels, equipped with teeny whips and wearing jockey caps. The camels were once ridden by little boy jockeys, but the system was phased out after protests of their ill treatment. "These robots are built on a Black and Decker drill," our driver tells us.

"How do they know what to do?"

We learn that there's a jockey inside the car, riding along with the owner and his companions, who controls the robot remotely. A walkie-talkie transmits his voice commands to the camels.

The radio announcer narrates in a steady staccato. "In the second place, Mohamed bin Ahmad bin Saed bin Houlu arrives, with Mazaal advancing to the second place, while in the third place we find Shaheen Hamad bin Ali bin Hafez al-Wahebi. In the fourth place, Al Shaare al-Ramhawi is advancing now."

The camels lope gracefully around the track as the remote-control jockeys urge them on. At first their lips flap complacently. But as the race progresses, a hidden competitiveness emerges. White foam flies from their lips, their necks stretch out long and flat, and they move into a gallop. We're hitting forty, then fifty kilometers per hour, flickering to sixty (about thirty-seven miles per hour), if I'm reading the speedometer right.

Our driver gestures to me to keep my head down. I realize it's not forbidden to have a woman in the car, but it's not the done thing either.

The commentary continues, minute after thrilling minute. "*Yasalaam, yasalaam, yasalaam* [joy], how wonderful, how wonderful, how wonderful and fantastic, and with Rahi, and with Rahi, Hamad bin Ahmad bin…al-Khouail advancing…"

The SUVs move in a fluctuating pack, their drivers skillfully avoiding collisions as we follow the high-haunched camels. *I could do this forever*, I think.

The announcer's tone intensifies. "Look at the final meters, look at the fantastic challenges, now look at the entry, the finish line, victory!"

Finally it's over, and we peel away from the track. The race lasted maybe fifteen minutes, but I wish it had never ended.

We leave the fairground for a nearby highway. I think we're going to stop for lunch, but the driver says, "Souk." We take a smaller road up a rocky rise, where camels are tethered near weathered white tents.

It's a Bedouin camp. Some people have brought their camels to the festival today, he says. He drives slowly along the dirt road. Women and little children sit outside tents selling plastic bottles of water, juices, and other items on small tables. The women's face coverings, resembling masks, give them a hawklike appearance. Called *battoulah*, among other names, the coverings date from pre-Islamic times. They are made of leather or gold fabric and tied on with cords. With a band around the forehead, they reveal the eyes but cover the lips. I've seen older women wearing them in the malls. Signifying maturity and marriage status, they are intended to conceal women's beauty. They also offer some protection from sun and blowing sand.

Behind the women and children, open tents, glinting with silver fabric and colorful strings, display camel harnesses and ties. One seems to be a kind of hardware store. Three stripped-down all-terrain vehicles are offered for sale outside, while cookers, tin boxes, tea servers, towels, men's jackets, and a roll of AstroTurf cram the interior. I spot a small tiger hide, with a crude half head and upper body without a taxidermist's artifice. It makes me uneasy. "Is this real?" I ask Tony and the driver, but we don't know.

It strikes me that this souk's not that different from old country stores that dotted the hollers near our farm. I'm happy that beyond Dubai's glamorous halls there's a place for these working families.

We head to the Camelicious farm to sip some milk and say our goodbyes, then pick up some camel milk chocolates for my son. I feel certain I'll be back for meetings about our autism clinical trial, and I hope it will be soon.

But just before we leave, I get a call — there's been a twist. A territorial brouhaha has caused a rift. Someone saw the media reports and felt left out of the process. Jutka's and my hoped-for camel projects must wait for another time.

I feel some grief for our project. Two steps forward, another step back: that's how the camel milk movement seems to go. But my work will continue, and I'm grateful for the inspiration. I board the aircraft and depart the desert, but it will stay in my spirit forever.

21 CAMEL MILK IN THE NOBEL LAB

"It's worth looking into."
— Dr. Jay Gargus

Newly back from Dubai, I attend a dinner at the University of California, Irvine, where Walid first sold camel milk. I've been invited by Dr. Jay Gargus, a pediatric geneticist and professor of physiology and biophysics, whom I met at an autism event. He'd caught my attention then because he said he was trying to cure autism, something you never hear from the medical establishment. He and his research team are doing some novel work.

When he asks what I've been doing lately, I tell him why I was in Dubai. "Camel milk?" he says. "I've done some work with mouse milk in autism." Now this is a man who speaks my language. "We had a child with a rare form of autism, with no known treatment. But experiments showed that mouse breast milk had tons of taurine, which helped mice with the disease. So I told his mom, just go down to the vitamin store and buy huge amounts of taurine. It's kept him alive, reversed lesions in his brain, and improved his behavior and seizures. Anyway, let's do something with camel milk here."

Amazing!

Soon we formulate a two-step plan. Step 1 will analyze some aspects of camel milk; step 2 will look for anything that might lead to an autism treatment. We'll compare camel milk with whatever milk I choose (to see how it's different, and as a scientific control). The laboratory where we'll do it was the site of research that won the Nobel Prize in chemistry. It showed how human-made gases used in aerosol sprays and refrigerants have damaged the earth's atmosphere and created the ozone hole. One of the Nobel team scientists, Dr. Don Blake, will help us out.

Dr. Blake, head of the chemistry team, writes me: "We are very excited to do this." For both doctors, this will be a "fishing expedition," as Dr. Blake says there's very little work on examining the gases given off by milk.

Why is analyzing gases important in medicine? He points to diabetes as one example. A person with severe, untreated diabetes lacks the insulin needed to process sugar and starts burning body fat instead. One of the byproducts of this process is acetone in the breath. "It's a gas. That smell was an early detection method once used by doctors," back when diabetes was a death sentence.

Such gases are known as volatile organic compounds (VOCs), explains Dr. Gargus. In the case of the child who was helped by taurine, VOCs detected in the child's urine were the clues that helped researchers identify the problem. "His body was making too much GHB [gamma hydroxybutyrate], which built up and became a poison to him." Because of its powerful sedative effects, GHB is used as a recreational and a date-rape drug.

This child's condition was accompanied by oxidative stress, resulting from an imbalance between free radicals in the body (from both the body's metabolism and external sources), and the antioxidants that normally keep them in check. Oxidative stress impairs the function of the mitochondria, components of our cells that produce energy and contribute to development. It can lead to chronic inflammation and may trigger a range of diseases, including forms of autism. In our experiments, Dr. Gargus will look for anything unexpected in the VOCs from camel milk, including components that might reduce oxidative stress.

Suddenly I seem to be codesigning an experiment.

My first thought is to compare camel milk with human milk,

because the two are often described as similar; but I don't know any nursing mothers I could ask to provide samples. And there are reasons to look closely at cow milk. For children around the world, cow milk, whether fresh or processed into infant formula, is by far the most commonly consumed type of milk, and children with autism and others frequently have intolerances to it. So I propose comparing both raw and pasteurized milk from cows and camels.

For analysis by their ultrasensitive lab equipment, the samples we use should be in top shape, as "udderly fresh" as possible. So whose milk should I use? Right away I think of Marlin. He lab-tests his milk with high-quality results. He has nice barns (where only religious music is allowed; that has no bearing on my decision, but it reflects his caregiving and just makes me smile). As I call him, I relish the fact that a man with an eighth-grade education will contribute to a piece of advanced scientific analysis.

After a few suspicious questions — what's this all about, and who's going to get the results — Marlin agrees. I also ask farmer Sam Hostetler and Meghan Stalzer of Mudita Camels, who apprenticed in Marlin's barns, to contribute samples.

When the boxes of milk arrive, I load them into the car and head for Dr. Gargus's lab. It's strange to park at a UCI medical building without Jonah in my arms, needing books and snacks. Dr. Gargus comes out to help me unload. Tall, he talks quickly and moves even faster. Even his emails are peppered with ellipses, like he ran off in midthought. He carries my boxes upstairs into a lab that looks like a mechanic's garage from thirty years ago.

I meet the other team members: Dr. Blake, a friendly, graying man, and Rafe, a thirtysomething guy with an endearing smile, reflective of his matter-of-fact personality and Down syndrome. Rafe assists by carrying boxes and doing other chores. Charlie, a young female graduate student, completes our group.

I open the box from Michigan, and there's Marlin's milk, packed like a dream: three fresh bottles of milk on one side, and bottles of colostrum (the first milk a mother expresses after birth, full of additional nutrients) and kefir (cultured milk) on the other.

Next we open Sam's box. The milk is frozen. I'd sent instructions to send it fresh. I guess he's not one for reading.

"It's okay, it won't affect what we're looking for," Dr. Gargus reassures me, seeing my somber face.

Meghan's milk didn't arrive.

Charlie explains the experiment's setup to me. "This is the bubbler," she says, indicating a glass tube and metal contraption. "The air inside will be vacuumed out. Next, we'll inject the milk into the tube and bubble helium through the milk sample, then collect the air that comes off the milk."

"What will that tell us?" I ask.

Dr. Gargus explains, "The air will contain the VOCs, small molecules that come from the milk." Each sample will yield only a minuscule quantity of VOCs. Charlie teaches me how to inject camel milk into the glass tube, using a tiny needle.

Meghan's milk arrives late the next afternoon. It wasn't frozen or packed in ice, so the lab can't use it. "Don't drink it," I tell Tony.

"It'll be fine," he says. He flash-pasteurizes it on the stovetop and drinks it all week, grinning every time.

A few days later I return. "So what are your findings?" I ask in the conference room where we meet.

Dr. Blake leans forward in his chair. "We saw a difference in the Michigan and Missouri milk. One of them had a lot of chloroform. Huge amount of chloroform. I mean, a scary amount in my book," he says, laughing and putting his hand over his heart.

"Scary for humans?" I ask. "Or just in gas or atmosphere terms?"

"In the old days, we used to use it to knock you out," says Dr. Gargus, miming a soaked handkerchief over his mouth.

"So where did the chloroform come from, and what does it mean for the milk?" I ask.

"One of my students found out that dairies tend to sterilize things with chloroform," says Dr. Blake. "It could be as simple as that. I'm positive that was nothing to do with the camels." *Good*, I think, because we don't need old Hollywood movie knockout drugs to mess with our results.

"So, from a single sample, one day's work: my team did not see anything that jumped out. We overlaid the chromatograms of cold raw camel and cow milk, and the VOCs looked the same, only with slightly different sizes," says Dr. Blake. "But we only looked at things small enough to vaporize into the lightest gases at cold temperatures. We didn't warm the milk, and that could have changed things. So this doesn't mean there is no difference between cow and camel milks."

"So, what did you learn by this first step, Dr. Gargus?"

"Comparing the VOCs — hydrocarbons, halocarbons, sulfur, nitrogen, oxygen compounds — in this camel milk, none of them showed as statistically different from raw cow's milk," he says.

Now for step 2: "Would differences in those things mean anything to you about autism?" I ask.

"Sure. The science community has no confirmed 'markers' to identify autism, so I can only try to search for things that might treat it. And I didn't see anything new. If we'd seen compounds that might mitigate oxidative stress, like the taurine in mouse milk, that would have been interesting. But that's an amino acid, and this test didn't analyze those," says Dr. Gargus.

But still, we've barely scratched the surface.

"Ninety-nine-point-nine percent of what's in the milk is in liquid form. We would need liquid chromatography machines to examine that, which means sending the work to another lab," says Dr. Blake. The researchers explain that we haven't examined the milk's antibodies, hormones, enzymes, fats, or other proteins, including the insulin-like proteins that camel milk may contain.

"So if this was archaeology, and the milk was an ancient midden heap, with layers of clue-filled garbage, we've only examined the very top one, and none underneath," I say. Dr. Blake agrees.

We lean back in our chairs. For me, there's more to discuss.

"So, just speculating, what's therapeutic in camel milk? Could it be the fat?" I ask.

"I don't know. We could do the analysis, but it costs a lot. I must tell you, if I put in a grant to the NIH to study camel milk, I —"

Dr. Gargus hesitates, "don't think you can get that funded." We laugh at his efforts to be delicate.

"And if we did those other things you didn't look at?"

"Is it worthwhile to analyze it? It sounds like 80 percent of camel milk is sold to parents of kids with autism," says Dr. Gargus. "While I'm sure you're largely responsible for that, obviously there is some pull." He's referring to my articles, videos, and lectures, but as he says, people keep buying it because they think it works.

"There's some research on using it for other conditions, like diabetes and celiac disease," I say.

"I don't believe there's something magical in it, so I think there's something we can measure. It's worth looking into," says Dr. Gargus.

"Anything to measure beneficial bacteria, that may affect our bodies' whole systems, as in the microbiome gut-brain concept that science is becoming aware of?" I ask.

"I would not know how to even start that," he says. "Bacteria produce jillions of compounds."

"Is it like asking you to analyze the universe? Bacteria's effects on the brain?"

"It is just too big. If it is *in* the bottle, we can figure it out. If it involves how the bottle changes stuff inside the kid's gut — *whoa.*"

"What would be the next place to look for differences from cow milk?" I ask.

"It would require investigating some very complicated protein function — maybe something signals the gut to do something different. Boy, you are getting into very fancy protein sequences, wow."

"Knowing that some people theorize an anti-inflammatory effect in camel milk, what do you think would be a mechanism of action?"

"You have to look at the functions of the different proteins there. You are waaay outside my domain of comfort," Dr. Gargus says, his face squinching like he's preparing to eat something sour.

"It could be a protein that's different, that metabolizes and gives off some gas, that goes into the gut, then into the brain — it's like the scientific metaphor of the butterfly that flaps its wings in Japan and we feel it here," muses Dr. Blake.

"It is a huge project...a very huge project," says Dr. Gargus.

"We could take this on if we had a staff person with a biochemistry background, at around a hundred thousand dollars a year, if you know anyone who can fund a grant. They would have to be anchored in a field that's able to survive attacks from less enlightened minds," Dr. Gargus adds, referring to camel milk's novelty in American science. "We wouldn't want this young person to stake his whole career on it — it might not leave him a place to go after that," he adds hastily.

Dr. Blake nods, and reminisces about their famed ozone-hole experiments, noting that the lead scientist, Sherry Rowland, was attacked incessantly by chemical manufacturers until he won the Nobel Prize.

But I don't have a hundred thousand dollars. And if I did, to keep up this chase, I might need a million dollars more.

"Thanks, gentlemen. You have both enlightened and depressed me," I say.

My conclusion? The benefits of camel milk could and should be further explored by analyzing the gases and also the properties of the milk in its liquid state. Camel milk, like autism itself, remains a puzzle for now.

I have to call Marlin to tell him about the chloroform the lab found in his milk. "What's that? You mean coliform?" he asks. Coliform bacteria are found in human and animal digestive tracts, as well as in air, water, and soil. It's legal to have a small bacterial count in milk, but Marlin's lab tests show that his is free of contamination.

"No, *chloroform*."

"What is this?" He has never heard the word.

"It's a chemical. They used to put people to sleep with it by putting it on a cloth and making them breathe it."

"Well, this lab must have made a mistake!" He's laughing but doesn't sound amused.

"No, they didn't. They have a very sophisticated lab."

He mulls this over silently. I hate delivering bad news to a man at dinnertime, especially one with a fractured hip (he got injured on his farm).

"So you think it's probably the cleaning stuff?" I ask.

"Maybe."

I inform him we didn't find any special markers in this experiment. "There's no real study. They won't be publishing anything. That would take too much money and time."

"Why not?"

"They said it would take more scientists and equipment. If I have a hundred thousand dollars they will. You have to have money to do science."

Again, the ways of the world are driven home to Marlin. It sounds very cold and conspiracy-theory-ish to pay for the science you want done. And I mentioned that the scientists had done this work with some leftover grant money from NIH (the National Institutes of Health), a federal agency, which probably spooks him. But he says nothing, and I say good night.

He calls back in thirty minutes. "Can you just check that it wasn't coliform, instead of chloroform? Maybe you don't know what you actually heard."

I hold the phone and play a clip of Dr. Blake explaining. We hang up.

He calls back again. "Am I keeping you awake all night, Marlin?"

"Mystery solved," he says. "The likely thing is the bleach. It could have been I didn't rinse as much that day because I wanted everything as sanitary as possible. Plus I had a freezer line bust and maybe it wasn't aired out. I'm going to bed. No reason to talk about it any more." I can hear the relief and satisfaction in his voice.

I won't give up on science, but I'm moving in a different direction. I'm headed to a place that looms large in the American imagination. Billed as the antithesis of everything deemed foreign, it shares some traits with Middle Eastern countries. It's the camel-speckled territory called Texas.

22 DOUG BAUM'S WORLD OF CAMELS

"Why wouldn't it be simple? This is a culture."
— DOUG BAUM

The road from hip and wealthy Austin to minuscule Valley Mills narrows to a single rugged lane. After speaking at a conference, I drive for two hours and park on a driveway made of dirt that turns to mud in every rain. Five mewling infant kittens circle me on shaky paws. American farms have unifying features: dirt, animals, denim, farm machinery, and truck parts. But this farm also has camels, a miniature Brahma bull, and a tiny donkey.

Doug Baum is outside waiting for me. "Hey, stranger!" he says. Just as I was instantly comfortable with Doug when we met at the second camel clinic in Ramona, I feel at home again now.

Built in the 1880s, the white Texas farmhouse feels smaller than it looks. Camel statues, blankets, Egyptian tapestries, and pieces of equipment festoon the living room. It has a warm and friendly atmosphere. The dining room window frames the camels a few yards away. The animals are the center of the family's lives. Doug's wife and three teens enjoy the camels and keep the farm running when he's away.

A fortysomething redhead burned pink by the sun, Doug normally wears head-to-toe khaki or a historical Union Army uniform. The khaki is for Egypt's Sinai Desert, where he leads tours among Bedouin communities. The blue uniform is for his role as a US Army Camel

Corps reenactor: the army had bought camels from Tunisia, Egypt, and the region that is now Turkey to use for transport before the Civil War killed the plan. Although Doug, a former professional musician turned zookeeper, didn't get a college degree, he knows a lot about history. He makes a living trucking his camels to church Nativity scenes and schools, reenacting the army's camel experiment, and doing camel treks and tours. Show him a camel saddle, and he'll tell you the country and era it comes from.

A gentle, patient man, he's learned much about camels and holds strong opinions about them. "Your camels are fat and lazy," I heard him tell a group of American cameleers. "They don't need all that food, or to drink all the time, or that equipment. All you need is this," he said, dangling a single rope.

We cross the wet grass toward a small, gently spinning windmill. A half-dozen camels with rain-dampened hair hang out in the paddock, lined up with their butts facing us. A white camel with pepper-brown tufts walks up to Doug. "Vergie!" His hands wrap her soft nose, the lines on his fingers furrowing as they kiss. She pushes her lips forward ardently. "Aww, look at her," says Doug. Her eyes close, and she takes two steps past him, raising her head dreamily. "See?"

She thrusts her back leg against his hand, her tail swishing like a broom.

"She wants you to milk her," I say.

"That's right. Vergie lost her baby a year ago — her first, a stillborn. We did our best, but what you can do?" he says, momentarily somber. "She gave milk for three weeks, around two and a half cups twice a day. We fed her alfalfa hay and corn, and the milk had the richest, sweetest taste. We put her back on the normal hay diet, and next day, my son took a drink and immediately declared the milk salty."

Vergie shoves her spread hindquarters against Doug, pushing him three steps back in his tall rubber boots. He grins. "We never have a lick of trouble out of her, and we never will."

As birds make "wheet, wheet" sounds around us, a male camel comes over to assert his status. Richard, at age eighteen, still has the blond majesty that spurred Doug to adopt him as a two-year-old. "He was the only male in a lot of four. Anybody with a brain would have taken the three females and started a dairy business, but he walked up and introduced himself. How could I say no to *this*?" Richard's brown ears match a patch on his nose. I stroke the underside of his anaconda-thick neck, ridged with hair. "This guy's toned. He's built," says Doug. Richard has appeared on TV shows, but he's also a star of Doug's Texas desert treks. He can go much farther than the twelve to twenty miles a day that paying human guests can handle, getting his only moisture from prickly pears and grasses.

Doug cushes Richard in the hay-strewn dirt, and I climb up. Sitting behind his hump, my knees slightly raised, feels like straddling a warm mountain. He rises in two motions, and my world falls and lifts. The dampness of his hair seeps through my jeans as we tour the paddock. I feel sky-high, grand as a princess in a medieval procession, impervious to bullets or distractions from below. I feel almost abandoned when he gently stops and cushes to let me off.

I know that camels aren't always as sweet-tempered and calm as Richard, so I ask a question. "Doug, is the mean, spitting camel true or a myth?"

"Camels spit, camels spit, camels spit," says Doug sardonically. "Hollywood has beat this idea into the ground. But they don't. They puke." He scratches Richard with two farm-roughened fingers.

"There's never been a camel in the history of the planet that just looked at somebody and said, you'll do, and then *pwuut*," he says, making a spitting sound.

"So they throw up?"

"They chew cud. If they get nervous, that cud comes up involuntarily. So my advice is, just don't make 'em nervous." He smiles slowly, enjoying himself. I shudder, hoping never to see it. I don't want to wash cud from my long, curly hair. Then again, maybe it's a good conditioner.

After a Bedouin-style dinner served with flatbread on round platters, I head off to sleep in Doug's small garage bedroom. The bed looks comfortable, but a black, thick-bodied spider menaces my feet. I grab a shoe to hit it, and it scrambles under the bed. I sneak into the house and lie on the living room sofa, where a stuffed animal head seems to watch me toss and shiver all night. A Texas-size lightning storm rolls in, and rain comes through the open windows. They say the state's latitude is the same as Egypt and perfect for camels, but right now it's damn hard to believe it.

The next morning is cold as hell, windy and gray. After breakfast, I look under the bed. The spider is still there. But I put it out of my mind, because Doug's taking me for a ride.

"I love a truck with busted bugs on it," I say, climbing into the cab behind his splattered windshield. We drive the green-gray grasslands of central Texas, past the hackberry, oak, and juniper trees fringing the road. Camels love to strip off the junipers' salty bark, he says, helpfully killing the invasive, water-stealing tree.

"See that bluestem grass? It's close to an Egyptian grass my buddies stuff saddle pads with. I chop a few clumps with a machete and make a saddle pad, nice and soft against the camel's body." He sells the pads with camel saddles he carries home from Egypt. "But instead of some Bedouin piece of wood from the trail, I use modern fasteners. It'll be good for the next three hundred years. Fifteen hundred bucks gets you the saddle, a pad, and all the bling a young camel guy would want," Doug says.

As he talks, I realize how deeply camel culture has permeated him. Though he lives in Texas, he relishes the minimal lifestyle of South Sinai Bedouins, including his "adopted family" in Egypt. "One pot for milking, cooking, and eating. One rope for camel handling and lashing bundles. One stick for walking, herding, and digging. One teapot, probably unwashed. Why carry two pots?"

They cook for him the way he cooked for me: "We have rice or pasta. Fresh Bedouin bread, like a tortilla. Fish, lamb, goat, or chicken. Vegetables. Hot brown Kool-Aid, we call it, which is about sixteen handfuls of sugar and a bit of tea. Breakfast is boiled eggs, jam, and bread with a block of sesame paste, like peanut butter." In the Muslim tradition, they eat with the right hand and regard the left as unclean (it is used for cleaning after elimination).

Despite the stereotype, not all his Bedouin friends like the nomadic way of life, he says. "There's always talk about setting them up in villages. The women really want that. A water source, that's the most important thing to them."

Doug's Bedouin friends are from the large Mezzina tribe, which migrated to Egypt from Saudi Arabia about four hundred years ago for better grazing, he says. Most Arab countries are run by peoples of Bedouin origin: the Hashemites of Jordan, Saudi Arabia's House of Saud, the Emiratis of the UAE, he adds. His friends, Sinai Bedouins, are ethnically different from the urban Egyptians who've lived along the Nile for nine thousand years, to his knowledge.

"How do they feel about camels?"

"The camel to the Bedouin is like the horse to the Western cowboy. Like in Western cowboy arts, the camel is glorified in poetry and songs. The Arabic word for camel is *jamal*, from *jamil*, meaning 'beauty.'

But even this beloved animal is kept in its cultural place.

"Virtue or beauty is given to camels in their names," he says. "But you tend not to see proper names, or names like Abraham or Jesus. It would be disrespectful to the prophets, because an animal is a low and dirty thing."

Doug fell in love with camels working a day job at the Nashville Zoo between music gigs, and then headed for Egypt to learn about them.

"I was instantly smitten. I had no knowledge, so I started hanging out with Bedouins in Sinai. On that first day, to kneel the camel for loading, they looped a rope to hobble the left foreleg, then passed the rope over the body so the camel felt it and stayed down. Super simple, super practical. There were dozens of these palm-to-forehead moments, and then I realize, why *wouldn't* it be simple? This is a culture."

Each Sinai Bedouin family owns camels if they can afford them. "Some don't have one anymore due to the drop in tourism. When I didn't understand the social dynamics, I'd ask horrible questions, like, Why do you only have one camel? And of course, the practical answer would be, If we have two, we have to feed two."

Young boys start working with camels around age four. "It's not a rite of passage, just part of their lives from the get-go. It's beautiful to watch. Nine- and ten-year-old boys know more about camels than I ever will." Girls help too, but not for long after puberty.

Strong male camels are preferred for work — there's no such thing as an untrained camel. Females are kept only for milk. "The Bedouins love to drink camel milk. They call it the natural pharmacy." Doug has been to an Egyptian camel-breeding farm near Birqash where they give free milk to sick people. "The man asks where I'm from. I tell him. He says, 'Oooohh, America…Egypt,' and puts his fists together in the international sign for brotherhood. I ask the man how his work makes him feel. 'It makes me happy to help people who need camel milk to be healthy. It's not a gift from me, it's a gift from my God,' he said."

But if struggling Bedouin families can't feed a camel, there's no milk for them or others in need.

"So what's the outlook for Bedouins, Doug?"

"If modern governments can settle them in housing, they can tax them. That's the whole point. But Bedouins are nomads, and tend to be a borderless people, so their allegiances are in question. For a generation, Sinai was Israeli-held. Through three wars, in Egyptians' minds the Bedouins were politically aligned with Israel, whether they were or weren't. When Egypt took over, the Bedouins were thought 'suspect' by the Egyptian government. There's still that distrust."

"In other words, they don't know what will happen?"

He looks grim. "They don't have a hand in their fate."

We return to the farm, where camels and kittens flick their tails in the waning light. Many domestic hungers are waiting to be satisfied. Doug pulls his rubber boots back on, strides to the paddock, and kisses an inquisitive camel's nose before reaching for the hay. "It's a great life. Wouldn't trade it for anything." Probably neither would his camels. They and Doug are crazy about each other.

I say goodbye and fly home to California, where some iconic camel lovers want to share their special culture.

23 THE MOST CAMEL-CRAZY COUNTRY IN THE WORLD

"Good luck with that."

— FEMALE SOMALI HERDER

My body is slowly sweltering in a San Diego apartment, but mentally I'm in Somalia. Just two hours' drive south of my Orange County home, it's like a different country. This tall concrete apartment block resembles a desert dwelling. Balconies rise around the courtyard like a step-well shimmering with water. It's home to my friend Abdi. In his early forties, he's a tireless father, community activist, cabdriver, and home health aide. (Somalis keep the local home-nursing and taxi communities going.) Abdi, tall and gregarious, is always eager to talk and help his people. I met him through Gil Riegler when Abdi was looking for camel milk. Knowing of my interest in camels, he's invited senior Somali community members to share their lore, but he's not sure if the elders will show up.

Somalia is the most camel-centric culture in the world. Located on the Horn of Africa, to the east of Kenya and Ethiopia, it borders the Indian Ocean and the Gulf of Aden. Its name is thought to come from a combination of *soo* and *maal*, meaning "go" and "milk," the very essence of nomadic pastoralism. Somali social structure and lifestyles are so predicated on camels that they are rumored to have nearly fifty words for the ruminant they love. There's even an official state camel named Maandeeq (meaning "milk-rich she-camel"), a lovely animal daubed

134

in the powder blue of the national flag. Business and personal transactions, community standing, common sayings, measures of wealth, their very ideas of survival reflect their camel ethos. After a lifetime with camels and large families in Somalia's jungles and stony deserts, these elders are spending their later years among sidewalks and strip malls.

I step inside the three-bedroom apartment. A jumbled pile of shoes sits by the door. "Should I take mine off?" I ask.

"No worry, sister, just be comfortable," he says. But I remove them. Abdi's little girl toddles over, not sure what to make of me but not shy. His wife, Rahmo, sweeps in, wearing a colorful headscarf and floor-length dress, and says hello with a wide smile. It's clear she's in charge of her own life. She and Abdi make an affable, if harried, couple, trading off care of their four children between his multiple shifts at caregiving, driving, and advocacy work. She shows him the food she's made, its thick steam rising from the slow cooker, and leaves again.

"Have a seat, sister," says Abdi, pointing to one of the low burgundy and gold floral sofas. No paintings or art are displayed on the walls. The girl clambers up and curiously touches my crystal bead necklace, her round face adorable under shiny black ringlets. I play with her as we wait.

When I sat at a table under the hot summer sun at the Somali Festival two years ago, at Abdi's invitation, I was ready to talk about autism. He wanted to bring awareness of the disorder to his people, as rates of autism among US Somalis are rising. White visitors stopped by the table, but Somalis passed without a look. At the end of the day, eating a fragrant rice and meat dish Abdi saved for me, I asked him why. "Sister, your message was good. We Somalis have a word for something, like a shame." He pronounces a word that sounds a little like *chi-chi*. "To us, autism is considered like that word. We would not talk about it in the open. So just having you here was good, to make awareness. Believe me, the people saw."

Now Abdi beckons me to his computer. "See sister, I've been watching this movie." It's an old film on YouTube showing nomads on the move, the bowed ribs and ropes of their portable homes, cooking pots, and bags piled methodically atop a camel. "I show the kids, especially the boys, so they know where they came from. They need to have pride, and stay out of things that are not so good." I know he's talking about street life and possibly Islamist extremism. The little girl watches too, pointing at the camel. No signs of autism in her.

Finally the door opens. An unsmiling woman enters, wearing a red Somali dress with yellow-gold edging. From her weathered copper skin and dark hair touched with silver, I guess she's in her early to mid sixties. She and Abdi speak in Somali. We nod, and I thank her for coming. Abdi had my questions translated before I came, and most of the elders have gotten them. Abdi sets up his video camera, and she sits on an ottoman before me.

"What is your name?"

Her reply sounds like "Aturo Seribe Abdulai," but we don't catch the spelling.

"Is it a family name or has a special meaning?"

She speaks in Somali to Abdi. "Everyone's name has special meaning to them," he relays. Hah, she put me in my place. I like it.

"Can you face the camera?" I ask.

No, she will not. She and Abdi confer. "Only her voice, she is comfortable with." So the camera's on me while Abdi translates my questions and the gentle, slightly guttural words of her answers.

"*Ma ku soo kortay noloshaada Geel dhaqashadiisa?* Did you grow up around camels?" I don't know if the words are spelled perfectly, but it's what Abdi reads from the list of questions.

"Yes. I left Somalia in 1990, arriving in the US in 2005 after a time in Kenya."

"Did you help take care of them, or was that a boy's job?"

Slim and muscular, she sits up straighter on the ottoman. "Yes," she says. "Everything. I herded, milked, and slaughtered camels. We had as many as fifty. I didn't sell camel milk — it was for the family." I already know that selling camel milk is taboo in most camel cultures because it's traditionally given free to the sick.

"What is the wisdom about camel milk?"

"There are three terms for camel milk. *Day* milk is fresh milk. *Suusac* is 'twelve-hour milk,' soured for twelve hours after milking. *Karuur* is 'twenty-four-hour milk,' which sits longer and turns into butter. The family drinks it daily. Any leftover is saved for guests or anyone who walks in." Offering guests the family's best camel milk maintains social honor. "We drink as much as the camels produce."

Her voice is a little scratchy with age, but she's speaking with confidence. Her face and bearing epitomize pride, the honor of being a girl doing the traditionally male work of handling camels.

A round-faced man with large brown eyes walks in. Ali Artan, a forty-two-year-old civil servant and an MBA student, is here to help Abdi translate. She turns away slightly but continues with Abdi and me.

"How did you use camels?"

"I have used camel meat and milk. If you drink a lot of camel milk and the doctor tries to put someone to sleep for anesthesia, it doesn't work, no matter how much medication they give. It's not like one glass will do it, it's drinking it every day. Those camel herders who drink the milk every day or every other day, they show more resistance to the medicine that puts people to sleep."

"Did you use camel milk to treat sickness? What kinds?"

"If you have a cough, they get the fresh milk, boil it, with two or three stones in it or in a pot, and they give to the person and then it cures them. If someone has a broken hand, we get one he-camel, slaughter it for him only, so he can recover. We saw it, take a rest, meat, fat, and camel is reserved for him. The roast camel will last longer than cooked. In a fire they dry it, and store it in a place," she says. Before I can ask if *roast* means smoked meat, there's an interruption.

Several older men enter the apartment. As voices rise in greeting, she covers her face with her scarf.

"Hey, chicken with three legs!" the men call to Ali Artan.

"They call him that because seeing him is as rare as a chicken with three legs, which never happens, you know," says Abdi, smiling as he keeps an eye on his daughter. "Or square with eight corners, they are calling him now," he adds. "Same thing, we always tell our kids go find a square with eight corners, but there isn't one."

I remember the Wisconsin joke about a round barn: "Guy went crazy and killed himself in there." Why? "He was trying to find a corner to take a leak and couldn't." But I just nod and smile briefly to the neatly dressed elders.

"*Salaam alaikum*," we say to each other, roughly meaning "God bless you." I am not sure if I should shake hands or not. Abdi introduces me, saying, more or less, "The camel lady, she is a writer, she wants to know about camels."

When I sit back down, the woman has closed like a sun-deprived flower. Yet we press on.

"Very important is the urine of the camel," she tells me, trying to ignore the men. "When snakes or similar animals bite a person with their poison, we give the camel's urine to them."

"Did people live on camel milk for a long time without other food?"

"They can live as long as they want without other food." (This is what I've been hoping to verify.)

"What is your main feeling about camels now, being an expert and leader as you are? Do you miss them?"

She responds as formally as she has the whole time. "In closing remarks, the camel is the backbone of the pastoral society. Without it, there is no milk and meat, and some sort of transportation is needed."

"Do you have children?" I ask, wondering if a woman who'd managed to work with camels might have had a different fate.

"What do my children have to do with camels?"

She seems affronted.

"That just means more hard work," I tell her. She relaxes again. This, she gets.

"It's not as bad as you might envision — having too many kids and camels is not a bad thing, not like in the city where you have to chase a child 24/7. That's because we are a communal society."

"That's what I wish we had more of in America," I tell her.

"Good luck with that," she says smartly.

I smile.

"*Mashallah*," she says ("what God wills," an expression of acceptance and approval).

"*Ma garanaysaa Heeso ama Gabayo lagau amaano Geela?* Do you know any songs or poems about camels?"

"I'm not a singer."

"It's just words," I tell her.

"There is a song. A guy comes to visit the family, and they go to milk an older camel for him, and he says, milk me the one who is younger."

"How did he know?"

"From the sound of the milk when it came into the container."

But she is too reserved to sing it.

"That concludes the mothers' discussion," says Abdi.

She stands.

"Can you stay?" I ask.

"No, she will not," Abdi explains.

The men have changed the whole dynamic. Maybe she doesn't feel it's proper for her to be here. She leaves with a brief hard turn of the lips that I can almost call a smile. I'm glad a woman has been the first person I've met to say that camel milk alone can sustain life. A life giver verifies the life-giving properties of the milk — that's a wonderful outcome.

24 I AM A CAMEL BOY

"A maiden will not complain."
— Mohamed Ali Dad

Now I'm in a province of men. They settle on the floor and low sofas in their socks, showing no interest in the woman's departure. And what a fun group! Despite the personal hell they've experienced, moving from country to country after a civil war tore Somalia apart in the 1990s, they're dignified, well-groomed, and articulate, laughing and teasing one another. They wear the slacks and pressed shirts of American grandfathers everywhere. While many of the younger Somalis I've met are tall and slender with high, rounded foreheads, these older men are shorter, with more angular faces. I'm not sure whether this means they're from a different ethnic group or whether it's just normal variation.

The Somali people are of complex origin, with their multithreaded history still under discussion. They have a strong oral tradition and didn't adopt an official written language until 1972. Almost all are Muslim, and many speak Arabic (plus English or Italian, a legacy of Somalia's colonial past) in addition to Somali or a dialect. Many are hardworking pastoralists. Socioeconomic differences are less pronounced than in other places because goods are often shared with extended family members and larger clan groups. Living in apartments when they're used to large families must be jarring, I realize. And lonely.

The first man to speak with me is Mohamed Ali Dad. With silver glasses and gray hair under a porkpie hat, he's so eager to talk that he's answered my questions in advance. He hands me four stapled sheets of yellow paper, written in a fine hand.

"Anytime, grandfather," calls Abdi from the floor.

"My name is Mohamed Ali Adad," he says softly in English, with a slight lisp.

"It mean 'spring stream,'" says Ali Artan, who is translating now.

"With two *a*s in my language, but in my American documents, just one," he says, "so here I'm Mohamed Ali Dad."

He turns his round, expressive gray-brown eyes to me, hands on his knees.

"I used to be a camel boy," he says. A tiny smile curves his lips. "I drive the camels to grazing areas. They eat all kinds of thorny plants. They like to eat from tall trees, prefer lush green plants," he says, his hands gesturing upward. "In the dry seasons they eat dry fodder from the bush, in the rains they eat grass. I am from a nomad family. They are always on the move. If they have sufficient grassland they will stay, but if the grass is scarce, they set for a new place."

I look at his notes. He's written: "I had to guard the camels against predatory animals and thieves as well. Every nomad wishes to own camels in order to survive in the semidesert. Camel thieves are a real nuisance, usually stealing from remote locations not near their locality. They cause bad blood among herdsmen."

He continues to speak. "We stayed out all day and brought them home after sunset, milked them, and drank the milk."

I check his notes to see if he has elaborated. Again, the legend is validated: "Nomads who raise camels can survive on milk alone, and have since time immemorial. When I was a camel boy living with my nomad clan, I drank milk in the morning and survived on that all day long. I drank after sunset when they were brought to the fold. This milk was my main or staple food all my early youth and childhood."

This alone is worth the drive.

He says, "We sleep separately from them, but you have to be vigilant in case they go out. If you lose camels, it's hard to live there."

His written words also flow with life: "Camel's owner is a big shot. He has a big say and commands respect among his clan members. The owner of a hundred camels is a rich man."

"People drink camel milk themselves and collect it for guests," he says. "The guests' milk is called *marti*. Guests can come at any time, so you must have something ready to offer them. Nowadays most nomads prefer tea, but then it was just milk. Each house would drink some and then put it in a big vessel so there was enough for guests. If they don't come, they drink it themselves."

"When we get guests in the US," says Ali Artan, "you know they are coming, but in pastoral society, they are gate-crashers!"

"Yes, there's no phone booth to call from," I add.

"In our culture, guest has number one priority. It is a disgrace if your guest leaves in hunger," Ali Artan adds.

"It's a *shame*," says Mohamed Ali Dad solemnly. "Then it will go around." He moves his arm in a circle. "That man doesn't entertain guests, and it's bad."

"You give the best, but you don't want them to stay more than three days," says Ali Artan, laughing.

"In Islam, guests can stay three days and nights, and you are duty bound to care for them. But after three days, it's an excess. It's a hadith [a teaching]," Mohamed Ali Dad explains.

"When a young man got married, did he give camels to his bride?" I ask.

"In the countryside the bride price was in camels," Mohamed Ali Dad recalls. "And it depended on the bride. If she belonged to a royal or noble family, the price was high. Olden days it was up to one hundred camels." The price of a bride from a poor and obscure family was meager.

Blood money and dowry are both paid in camels, I learn. "If someone kills your woman, the blood money is fifty camels," he continues. "But if a man wants to marry a woman, it's up to one hundred camels. Camels are treasure trove. Camels and girls. We start a fight? We give gifts to the clan whose men were killed. They marry these girls and they have children with them. We solve all our problems with camels and girls."

Ali Artan, perhaps aware of how this sounds to my ear, gently says, "It keeps the peace. When people intermarry, you want to live in harmony as they are family, instead of a zero-sum game. But we are not as unlucky as the Maasai [East African cattle-herding nomads], who must kill a wild lion before they can get married. At least we can come up with one hundred camels, but I don't have to fight with lions," he says, smiling. "Good luck with that!"

"In South Sudan," recalls Mohamed Ali Dad, his eyes widening, "the bridegroom has to bring a live crocodile."

"Do they eat it?" I ask.

He doesn't know. "But it's a condition." And he had a wedding challenge of his own. "I met my wife in town," he says. "In town they deal in money. They make a price, and if it's too much" — he waves his hands up and down — "you negotiate. It's written, then two witnesses sign it." His city wife cost him the equivalent of ten camels. "I paid cash."

The baby girl cries, "Daddy!" She's getting fussy in this room full of men. I make a consoling face at her.

I look at what Mohamed Ali Dad has written. "Somali nomads rarely fall sick. They are slender and wiry, and you'll never see an obese nomad."

"Does camel milk make ladies slim and strong?" I ask. "I heard there was a nomad song about a woman, saying she's as slim and beautiful as a woman who has drunk camel milk all her life."

"Yes." His reply on the yellow paper says, "They are shapely and graceful, though may look skinny."

"Are there camel songs?"

"Yes. There is a song about a camel boy talking to his camels at the well." His hands shape a well. "He says, look, listen to me" — he shakes his long forefinger — "you are going to a desolate area, and you will stay without water for thirty days. So take enough water, take your fill *now*. Because you will be without water for one month."

"Is that how long they can go?"

"Yes, after one month you have to take them to the water."

"And if they don't get it?"

"They will suffer."

"How long will they go before they die?"

He looks perplexed.

"Usually the camel owners take them before they go. Because if the camel die, they die also. In Somali they say — " he speaks a soft, lyrical phrase.

I can see that letting a camel go without water is inconceivable.

The other men tell me Mohamed Ali Dad is well versed in history, so I ask: "Because you are a scholar, do you think people used camel milk and meat before Islam?"

"Islam came through Mecca, then our areas. The first people who took Islam after the Arabs were Ethiopians."

"So before Islam, what was the religion? A nature religion?"

"Somalis are Afro-Asian, and they had their own system," he says. "But I do not know what it was. Then Holy Islam came." This reminds him of another hadith. "Regarding camel urine, in my area, we never saw camels' urine as medicine, but the lady here [the woman I was interviewing] used it in her area. But in the teaching, if you mix camel milk and urine, it's a panacea, the word that means cure for all. And the Prophet says drink camel milk and use with the urine and drink. I never did have it, but I would try."

"I trust what the Prophet (PBUH) said," his notes read. "Whatever he said was a revelation and not from his own."

I've heard about camel urine as a therapy for cancer. But he won't get to try it back home, it seems: he's probably here to stay.

"I have never been back to Somalia," he says. "I came from the Middle East, in Saudi, then to the US."

He doesn't sound sad, but his words touch my heart. "They keep camels in Saudi, but the farmed milk is not the same as the camel that goes to the bush and eats and drinks from different trees. It should go to the jungle, feed on different plants. If you wish to drink camel milk, you look for the one who grazes outside. It's just like the honey. The bee that goes to the bush, their honey is more healthy."

He shifts toward me.

"Can you start a camel milk business?"

"I looked into it," I reply, "but it's not easy to do."

"Anybody who sells camel milk in America will be very rich," he says solemnly. "You bring them from Australia."

"Yes, but it costs a lot. If somebody has millions of dollars, call me," I tell him.

"It's time for a nice break now," says Abdi, his voice strong in the apartment. He places a tall golden teapot on a stack of carpets on the floor. The men stand and stretch, fetch plastic plates. We serve ourselves from the slow cooker. I copy the men, pinching up mouthfuls of spicy chicken and vegetable stew with small pieces of warm flatbread. I make sure I use my right hand.

As we relax, soft Somali words drop and float around me, like curled autumn leaves in a bubbling brook. The men's hands that once drove camels with ropes and sticks now fiddle with key chains and teacups. Their mellifluous voices rise and fall.

I have a surprise. I pull out a chocolate camel wrapped in gold foil. "It's from Dubai," I say. "We can all share." They look at the package as if they can't quite believe it.

"It's a camel?" says Mohamed Ali Dad.

"Yes, made with camel milk. It's hollow, like…" I was going to say like chocolate Easter bunnies. "It's not solid."

"Oh, we can eat camel now," says someone, laughing. I expect Abdi or I will break it open, but no.

Abdi gets a good-size knife and a plate. I set the camel gently on the piled carpets. The two Mohameds bend to watch. I peel back the foil, which is wrinkled artfully over the camel's body to resemble hair.

"We have to do this right, grandfather!" says Abdi.

They speak in Somali. Abdi turns the camel on its side. The knife is positioned at the neck.

"In the name of Allah," says Mohamed Ali Dad, and the little chocolate head rolls onto the plate. Cheers go up. The men settle on the sofas with pieces of chocolate. Abdi lies with his elbow propped on the carpet. "It's very good," the men say. They eat it slowly, puzzling over it. It's camel milk but yet it's not, their faces seem to say. But they're in a great mood.

I wonder if Abdi's little girl will ever taste camel milk. What will she miss?

"Okay, after this break of good rest and food, let us resume," says Abdi.

The imposing elder of the group has sat without addressing a word to me. He has a very dark, high-cheekboned face with a short silver beard above a striped shirt. His deep-set eyes and strong hands match his voice and radiate a sense of leadership. Salad Samatar is new to the United States. His name was mangled on arrival. "The government changed his first name to his last name! America is confused," the men joke.

"Tell him we are confused about lots of things," I say, laughing.

It's Salad's turn but he has already reengineered my structure. He tells Ali Artan in Somali that he only wants to answer questions others haven't. I quickly change my plan and ask the first new question I can think of.

"How does the Somali culture view the camel? Do they cherish it? Are they inspired by it? How do they feel about it in their heart?"

Ali Artan translates the question into soft Somali.

"To begin with, the camel is a priceless species. It gives milk, meat, and transportation. Beyond that," and passion fills Salad's voice, "if you are away from the camel, for a month it may not need anything to eat. It might be in the forest for a year without water except eating grass and plants." The green plants have moisture in them, he says, speaking only in his language. "And camel herders will drink only the milk for a long period of time, a year."

"Do they feel good living only on camel milk for a year?"

"No fruits, nothing else. And they feel good on it."

"What are your memories of camels, the lessons you learned?"

"Camel's milk is medicine." He stabs the air with his finger. "You reminisce. You will have flashbacks remembering that you miss it. When the person is sick, the milk is given to the patient with camel urine. It also helps the digestion system if they have constipation."

"Do you think it gives you diarrhea, like Saudis do?" All the men laugh.

"It's a flushing system, like taking your car to a car wash. It cleans the bad and takes it out," he replies.

"Kills the bacteria," Mohamed Ali Dad chimes in.

Salad does not look at me, only at Ali Artan, though he glances in my direction once or twice.

"When you look at the young kids here, do you see the difference?" I ask Salad.

"Don't you get it? They are missing the vitamins of camel milk! It's *obvious*." Salad's soft words are punctuated by popping sounds. "It's like comparing apples and orange. The camel boy runs faster, with no complaints. No 'I have a muscle pull out, I'm sweating, I can't run because I haven't gone to 24 Hour Fitness.' The camel boys are impromptu runners. These kids here, they have lots of problems! They try to run, soon after they are very tired, lazy. You cannot compare the camel boy with the San Diego Somali boys."

Mohamed Ali Dad interjects: "I am a camel boy. Guess my age!"

"Oh, oh," I say, laughing. "You are in great shape!"

"Throw a number!" Abdi says. "I start for you — forty-five."

"Sixty," says Ali Artan.

"Uh, sixty-five," I say hesitantly.

"I am seventy-nine. That's a camel boy."

"Your physique!" I say. My hands go straight up and down.

"Everything is perfect. Even a maiden will not complain."

The men erupt with laughter.

"I heard that too!" I say with a smile, confirming their explanation.

"She wouldn't complain," says Ali Artan, laughing but serious. "Maybe me she would complain," he jokes. "I'm forty-two. I would tell her, there's a timetable for everything! But not him. He is a camel boy. That is something you can't take away from him. His body is less fat, muscle is fit, as you can see."

"My father died in 2003 at maybe eighty-nine or something," Mohamed Ali Dad says proudly. "He was married at the age of twenty or eighteen or something. His children and their children now number over 110."

"That's a camel boy!" say the men.

"I am the eldest, the chief. I have eleven kids, eight grandkids, split between Somalia and the US," says Mohamed Ali Dad.

"A town boy who manages a wife and two kids, that is *his* limit!" says Ali Artan.

Salad has given me a very quick glance twice as the good humor grows.

"How many kids do you have?" I ask him.

"Everyone has kids," says Abdi kindly, as if explaining something simple.

Salad says he is a father of thirteen.

"In Somalia, how do you make money to support thirteen kids if you have camels?" I ask.

"I was a nomad and also lived in a small town."

Ali Artan clarifies, "People like this in a small town, maybe they have a small business or two families. People in the bush supply the cities — it's an economic supply chain. People need milk and meat, and pastoral people have those."

When the milk that keeps them fed is in short supply, nomads buy food from townspeople or slaughter a he-camel and eat its meat. She-camels are rarely slaughtered.

"The pastorals come to the small town for goods like sugar and salt," Abdi adds. "And so Salad lived in both worlds."

Mohamed Ali Dad throws out, "Everybody lives on milk. No bill comes to you. You have a nomad chief with four wives, everybody drinks the camel and goat milk. No bills to pay."

Ali Artan says, "No utilities! No rent, no T-Mobile. Cheaper than here!"

"Only food and clothing," adds Mohamed Ares, a scholarly-looking man with light-gray hair. Ali Artan says he's an accountant. He's been sitting on a chair by the window. Like the others, he seems to know a lot about Islam.

"You can sell or barter animals," says Mohamed Ali Dad.

Mohamed Ares says, "You can lend something from your neighbor and pay later."

"You can have a lot of wives and kids in Islam, right?" I ask Mohamed Ares.

"In Somalia you can have four wives, but you have to be equally fair to them in Islam. It's hard," he adds.

"It's hard," they all chorus.

"And that won't happen," say Mohamed Ali Dad. "So please, better keep one wife."

Ali Artan adds, "It means emotionally fair too, and people are only human, whether you are Christian or Muslim. It's not a joke."

Mohamed Ali Dad says, "Prophet Mohammed had nine wives. Aisha was the youngest. He *love-ed* her. He spoke openly about it. He says, 'Oh, Allah, I am trying to be fair, but you control my heart.'"

Mohamed Ares politely interjects, "May I add something? The Islamic teaching allows you to marry four. But you must offer fair treatment physically, economically, everything. So the last fifty years you will never find so many people with so many wives."

"Did it used to be more?" I ask.

"Because of your income, the rent, the way you live, yes," he says. "You will never find it now, with very few exceptions."

I have one more question. "Did anyone of you remember people who were mentally ill, or had autism, or cerebral palsy? Or kids who could not learn, or acted strange? Or could not walk well?"

They stare into space, thinking. "No," says Mohamed Ali Dad. "No," says Mohamed Ares. Salad shakes his head. Nothing like that.

"If someone broke a bone, we would kill a camel and he would eat it for forty days, and then he will get better," says Mohamed Ali Dad. "But no problems like that. Of the mind or body."

"No more video, sister," says Abdi. "We ran out."

The room has gotten as hot as a desert. Out of respect for their traditions, I'm still wearing a shirt over my sleeveless top, and my face is shining with heat. Abdi's face gleams too. But the elders have borne it with equanimity, like so much else.

We stand, chat, and laugh. Someone shakes my hand. Salad is

almost facing me now. He looks happy too. Thinking that he also wants to shake my hand, I hold it out. He loops my arm in his, as if we were square dancing, and gives a courtly nod. We never touch.

I say goodbye to Abdi. He's glad they came, and relieved at how the gathering turned out. "Everybody was happy to talk, sister."

Alone outside in the late-day sun, I see an outline of their country in my mind, an invisible Somalia floating in the air. I imagine the losses these people have endured — their camels, their loved ones, departed relatives lying under faraway stones. They see their descendants' health declining. Grief for them clouds my vision. I stand on the steps, trying to process it.

I'm just a bystander, far from understanding their ways. I haven't breathed their earth, tasted their food, heard their camels moan in the night. Some of their traditions for women aren't for me. But I honor the good from their culture. After all, they put up with mine.

Before I walk to my air-conditioned car, I read Mohamed Ali Dad's last handwritten page.

"I miss camel's milk and meat greatly. I long and yearn for them. I feel great nostalgia to my nomad simple life where one pays no bills and no rent and where one breathes fresh air. And where a man can marry a maiden whose bosom is equal to the size of a fist."

25 MARLIN TAKES A STAND

"I won't seek a political solution to a spiritual problem."

— MARLIN TROYER

"How's the weather? The post office says the mail carriers might not even show up in your area," I say during a phone call to check in with Marlin.

"That's the government for you," he says. He despises all things government. From his talk, you wouldn't expect him to be a peaceable man. Yet he's a pacifist by tradition, a volunteer emergency medical responder, and very community-minded. He's my friend now, but like a firecracker, he can explode in your hand.

Today, he's already done with his work and isn't concerned about the weather. "What health conditions are people using the milk for these days?" He knows, but he doesn't keep records on his customers' uses for the milk. I ask why not.

"Is that in case some Michigan authorities try to bug you?"

"No, I'm not too worried. You got two groups who support raw milk — the Constitution-loving, freedom-supporting guys like me, and the tree-hugging, greenie types. It's changing in this country, and they can't stop it for too long."

Then he makes a prediction. "As the population gets less God-fearing and more bold with deviant behaviors, there are now people who won't buy from me because of my opinions. I told my liberal neighbor, who is a total socialist and all rainbow gay marriage and such, you really enjoy me as a neighbor, but you are living two different lives. Most of the people in your camp would be happy to take my kids away from me, as I homeschool and teach what you view as extreme Christianity. We are like pets of society, and everybody oohs and ahs. But there will come a time when Amish and Mennonite will be classed as bigoted people and shunned for their beliefs on *homusexshality*," he says, probably pronouncing it that way since he doesn't watch mainstream television, isn't around people who casually use the word *sexual*, and would never think to ask gay people what they prefer to be called. He makes me laugh even as he pushes the limits of my indulgence. He might be right about this prediction, but maybe not. The mood of the country is turning left *and* right.

But he wouldn't take the actions some of his conservative non-Amish neighbors say they would, were their big-government fears to materialize. "I won't seek a political solution to a spiritual problem. There's only one right way to live," he continues. "The God of the Old Testament. Our country was founded on this. It's the only way a society can work."

"Is this the view of most Amish people?"

"No, because some just don't know about this kind of thing. I'm not your average Amish/Mennonite guy, because I'm highly interested in the larger world. But standing by to see the kingdom of heaven rule over the world? Yes, we have that viewpoint."

Marlin applies his morals to his tussles with Walid, who he sees as pushing the Amish farmers too hard. ("We are going to be very competitive on price," Walid had told me in a steely tone. "It is not a good time to be holding hands with Marlin.") Now the price he pays for their milk is going down.

Walid had posted a price discount on the Facebook customer group on a Sunday, an act that still stings Marlin. That's a day Marlin and the Amish reserve for worship. Marlin, the online defender of Amish farmers who can't access computers, viewed this as a price war "sneak attack." So he barred Walid from the group, but then they spoke, and he added him back.

"The Bible says, do not go with them — do not sit in the seat of the scornful," Marlin says. "Walid and I are still friendly. It's an issue of no longer collaborating with somebody that has demonstrated what he has." He's also referring to Walid's initial mislabeling of bottles as purely "grass-fed" milk and media comments Walid has made that he perceives as taking credit for Amish milking. But it's more than that. Marlin is focused on milk and serving families. Walid wants a product he can sell to get rich. They're as different as a ram and a leopard.

Adding to Marlin's worries is his fear that Walid is using camels to "bring jihad," or holy war, to America. "Those people don't want to give camel milk away to America, they want it to support their image and way of life." I'd scoffed at this, but since Walid is aware that such suspicions exist, I'd asked him about it. He is very religious and supports strict Saudi-style Islamic principles, but said he's practicing the form of jihad that is "struggle against the self to live a better life." I tell Marlin to lay that idea to rest.

Despite his mini-battle with Walid, Marlin serves people without regard to their faith, something all the camel milk vendors do. His website shows a cross next to an image of a camel, but he says his website designer added that without asking. "However, I don't think it's shameful to use my business as a witnessing tool. Myself and Walid are the same in that aspect. There's more to us than business — there's also a strong belief system."

"And beards," I remind him.

"Yes," he says, as if he'd never noticed before. "That's funny."

I adore how our camel milk community crosses cultural boundaries. It's united by its challenges and rewards. Fundamental and pastoral societies have habits in common (keeping women at home, avoiding mainstream schooling, maintaining ties to land and animals, being guided by religion). They're often not in step with liberal mores. But some of their perspectives add richness to modernized cultures, revealing strengths and weaknesses in both.

For instance, Marlin is vehemently opposed to milk pasteurization. I too prefer raw milk, because heat can destroy some compounds that may be beneficial. But in the interests of offering a nutritious, nonallergenic, risk-free food in places where raw milk can't be produced or stored safely, I'm not opposed to pasteurizing it. This he can't wrap his mind around. "I love you, but I don't *understand* you," he moans. In a perfect world, though, I would agree with him.

We also agree about the FDA's unhelpful attitude. Legalizing the interstate transport of raw camel milk would make suppliers' and customers' lives much easier. It could be justified on the grounds of compassionate use and its safety monitored by simple tests of farms and shipments. But the camel milk market is small, and the FDA would rather ignore it. I don't even bother trying anymore. The rules, as ever, favor financial and scientific powers. No one's interested in mothers or pastoralists.

I'm used to this: I've worked for the government. But it's enough to make an Amish camel farmer rant. Still, his mission is serving those who need this special milk. That's a fundamental belief I can support.

26 CAMEL CLASHES AND CULTURES

"It would be like saying, pray to your local supermarket."

— DR. RICHARD BULLIET

My cab zigzags through Manhattan as Mohamedou, the driver, dodges several anniversary ceremonies of the 9/11 terrorist attacks. A light rain drizzles on me as I enter the leafy green gates of Columbia University. On the high floor of an academic building, I find a camel oasis. Having seen how religious the camel cultures are, I want to learn more about the origins and importance of their beliefs about camels.

"I may be the only camel guy in Manhattan," says Dr. Richard Bulliet as I enter his book-lined office. An Illinois boy who "always had a talent for gathering collections of odd facts," he's studied the Middle East, religions, and camels since 1967. His smooth, blue-eyed, pink-cheeked face makes age seventy-three look good. I settle in the corner under a collection of camel statues.

"Why are you asking about camels?" he says, more statement than question.

"Have you heard of camel milk in the news, how it's helping kids with autism, like mine?"

"No. Not at all," he says firmly.

"That's what got me into this. So I want to know about their history and involvement in religions."

Resorting to his classroom habit, he begins at the beginning. Camels aren't even in the story yet, because he starts with asses.

"Do you know about asses' milk?" he asks.

"Heard of it, but not much."

"Asses' milk is mostly used in Northern Europe. It's regarded as having special value, but most of it's going into cosmetics."

"I'm mostly into camels and camel milk," I say. I feel panicky at having to learn about another weird milk, so I come back with a question. "Some people think Middle Eastern and African cultures venerate the camel, that it's almost holy. Is there a basis for that?"

He fixes his lecturer's gaze on me. "Islam has almost no overlap with camels. The culture was engaged in camels before Islam. Most didn't view them as special. They were a source of food, fiber, and labor."

"So they weren't worshipped or even given special esteem?"

"No. Most domestic animals don't have a mythic profile, although some do."

Cows, sheep, goats, and pigs were first domesticated in the Middle East and Egypt around ten thousand years ago, he explains. Cows were popular mainly in North Africa and Turkey. But people didn't really *use* these animals for another two to four millennia.

"So why the heck did people keep farm animals before they actually used them?"

"That's when mythology kicked in," he says. He gets very precise. "There are three stages of human-animal interaction: separation, when early humans became self-conscious and knew they were a different species. Then predomestication, when they start thinking about animals — animals enter art then, and language may describe them."

"So this was the age of animal myths?"

"Yes."

"What ended it?"

"Domestication. As we began using animals, they became largely despiritualized in our eyes. The philosopher Descartes called them inanimate machines."

This sounds sad to me. Spiritual practices across time have used animal symbols. The animal-human connection may have been primal, but seems mostly absent in today's religious landscape.

"When did people start using camels?"

"They appeared with traders from Sinai and Israel, around 300 BCE in Southern Arabia. In the Torah, Joseph was rescued by traders with camels."

"Did you see the scholars blasting each other in the news, when a new archaeological study said there were no camels in the Levant area in Abraham's day?" I ask him, smiling. This camel fight had theologians hyperventilating. The discovery implied that early Biblical accounts of camels were anachronistic and meant the Bible had gotten the facts wrong. The suggestion of fallibility in holy texts always triggers a fight.

"Eh," he shrugs. "Camels could have been encountered in trading between regions then, although they weren't common. But the thing to know is there was no real camel god. A caravan god represented traders, but camels were not venerated."

"So what about the Qur'an verses? 'Behold the camel, will they not look at the camel Allah has created, use it for your needs,' you know."

"Islamic hadiths about camels stressed their utility. The Prophet was basically telling his people to use the camel, not worship it."

"It was practical advice?" I ask.

"Yes. Basically saying, here's a good animal, use it. Otherwise it would be like saying, pray to your local supermarket."

Camels have always been relatively easy animals to manage, he says. "Since camels in deserts had no predators, they weren't very stress-able. So domestic camels *are* the wild camels, domestic-ready from the very start! Even in battle, camels don't startle. They'll take bullets and still lie down." By contrast, he says, wild Bactrians, the double-humped Asian cousins of dromedaries, "are very flighty today, but maybe they weren't always."

Even camel colors are affected by the issue of domestication. Different regions have different colors because of humans selectively breeding them, he tells me. "Whiteness in animals has a strong association with domestication. It's purely genetics. You can see it in rabbits and dogs. In Niger, the camel stock was so limited you could select for color, and they liked piebald."

However, since the spiritual significance of the camel is limited in his eyes, he returns to the donkey, which has a special importance in all the Abrahamic religions — Islam, Judaism, and Christianity. "Every messenger of God rides on a donkey," he says, and there's a tradition that all these donkeys are descended from the same sacred line. The donkey's holy reputation was also usurped by the "dark side": "In Islam, in the end times, the Antichrist rides a donkey, as a peripheral prophet. Then he gets killed with a spear."

But calling someone an ass was an insult even then. So why is the humble-looking donkey revered more than the majestic camel? "This whole importance of the donkey in religion is based on the prodigious size of its penis." He smiles. "It's legendary. Compared to donkey lore, the camel is barely a pimple. It doesn't amount to a hill of beans."

While I'm thinking what a buzzkill this is for Walid's worshipful camel-marketing message, I ask Dr. Bulliet for some background to better understand Walid and his feud with Marlin. After their clashes over pricing, treatment of farmers, sales techniques, and personality differences, their relationship has finally crashed. Richard is not surprised.

"The US and Saudi Arabia are the most similar countries in the world. They hate each other like cousins. Both are devoted to spreading the gospel. We like our religious doctrine the same way Saudi tribes like theirs."

I refer to Marlin's suspicion that Walid is "bringing jihad" to the US through camels, by which Marlin means a war on Christian faith. "So what does jihad actually mean?" I ask. "Does it mean struggle against self, like Walid says?"

"It can. That's higher jihad. 'Lesser' jihad is violent struggle to protect the faith."

"What do you think of a Saudi business owner dressing in Amish clothes to promote his product? How is that viewed in Islam?"

He shrugs and says, "It's nothing to him. Just another form of Western clothes. When you fly to Saudi Arabia, as the plane gets close to landing, the men on board change from Western clothing to the thobe and headdress — their cultural attire. It isn't religious garb. It doesn't have anything to do with Islam, it's just their national costume."

"Do you think Walid can run a camel milk business here, when he says he won't violate Islamic faith guidelines to borrow money or get a line of credit? And he shifts his story for investors so easily."

He shrugs again. "Your friend is pretty typical. Sounds like he was raised well, in a proper Islamic manner. Obfuscating things for potential investors wouldn't single him out among entrepreneurs. It's kind of standard operating procedure."

Our meeting ends as he gives me a copy of his latest book. Richard's knowledge of history has lent sparkle to my horizons.

27 WHAT KIND OF CRAZY THING IS NEXT?

"Camels seem like clean, motherly creatures."
— JONAH

When Jonah gets in my car after school, he puts the radio on hip-hop as a second choice — he prefers metal, but the kind I don't like. Now a high schooler, he sits tall in the front seat. His shoulders are large with muscle in his favored green plaid shirt, and his skateboarder's thighs spread wide over the leather. "Hey, Mom," he says. "How was your day?"

"Fine," I tell him, happy that he asks about me. It wasn't always like this — his perspective-taking skills have greatly improved. Neurotypical (aka regular) people can mentally put themselves in another's place and make the proper social comments, but for people on the autism spectrum it's often a skill that has to be learned. "You?"

"Pretty good. I'm doing great on my grades. Got two exams back, and I got As in art and history. I expect I'll do pretty well in English and social studies too." The ocean breeze coming through a rolled-down window ruffles his wavy light-brown hair.

"Great."

We bob our heads in silence. "We watched a movie about Gandhi today. He worked so hard for peace," he says. "But when he finally got his life's dream, after all he did to help India, the country split over religion."

"Yeah, Partition, when Pakistan was split from India. Lots of lives lost. Glad you're learning about that. I never did in school." While I've always educated myself on some issues of other cultures, I've learned the most about Asia and the Middle East through getting involved with camels.

"Yeah," he says. "It's just kind of sad. He did everything to make his vision come true, then it turned out the exact opposite."

"Sometimes that's how it works in life. Not often, though," I say, trying to reassure him. "You still have to try to make the world better."

Jonah's interested in politics and history, but mostly he's into humor. His activism is helping to clean up the beach. He's skilled at drawing, he can run a sewing machine, and he wrote a song that's worth publishing professionally. With all those voice lessons, he could sing in public — if he wanted ("That was your goal, Mom, not mine"). His life isn't perfect. He still struggles with organization, a few social skills, and getting chores and homework done. But he's doing amazingly well considering where he started. And he knows a little about how he's helped people through my first book and the camel milk movement. Everything I've done is because of him — he's an indelible part of my being. I just want other kids to have the chances that he did.

We drive comfortably past the store where I bought the dress to marry Tony, in a wedding where Jonah escorted me down the aisle and we shared a mother-son dance. We pass the intersection where I once waited at a red light and thought desperately, *There is no place for us.* Now, as I relax in the flow of his talk, I recall that night, and briefly wonder how we survived.

Driving along, I come out of my reverie. "Darn it, I missed my turn. I accidentally headed to our old house, honey," I say.

"That's okay. Just make a right on this street. It'll get us to the new place."

"Hey, guess what?" I throw out, deciding to share the weirdest news of my day. "Looks like donkey milk is helping people too. It's being used in hospitals for babies who can't handle the other milks, like soy, cow, and nuts."

"Oh, really?" he says with interest.

"Yeah. That part about babies in hospitals being given camel milk was the first thing I ever heard about it. So maybe donkey milk works the same as your camel milk."

"Donkey milk?" He thinks it over. "I don't know…"

"Really? Why?"

"Camels seem like clean, motherly creatures. But donkeys…they sound unhygienic. Kind of creepy to think about, actually."

"Plus they only have two teats and give about a liter or quart a day," I add.

"Hmm, not much," he says. "And where do they even have them? Most people don't own them here."

"Italy. I don't know where else. It's not likely to be on the market anytime soon."

"Guess not."

The next day I'm asked to join a Facebook group called Healing with Donkey Milk. A farm has started in America. My way lies with camels, not donkeys, but I join and start to read. Someday a child might need this "crazy" milk, and I want to be ready for that plea.

28 INDIA REDISCOVERS ITS TREASURE

"My child has autism."
— INDIAN OFFICIAL

From my room in a high-rise Mumbai hotel I look down at the Queen's Necklace, a long curve of lights sparkling on the shore of the Arabian Sea. The soft, blue-gray sky holds seagulls and clouds. But monsoon season has just ended, so there won't be rain. Flying through the night from New York felt like time travel. This sleek, glass-walled room is entirely modern and nontraditional: no embroidery or Mughal arches, only blond wood and white sheets. The only color comes from an apple, lying round and red in a bowl. But tomorrow I journey to Rajasthan, where the camels wait. As my work and writing about camels and their owners have expanded, I've been invited here to raise awareness about the benefits of camel milk.

In Jaipur, the state capital of Rajasthan, I head from the plane to a TV station, where I slip into a new stiff pink *kameez* (tunic) sparkling with rhinestones and a matching *dupatta* (scarf). The *churidar*, or leggings, ruche properly around my ankles, resembling the *churi* (bangles) they're named for. Indian friends had suggested I wear local clothing so that people would feel more comfortable and happy that I appreciate their culture. This is great, as the clothing is beautiful, yet practical to wear. Some men politely lead me to a polished studio, where a screen shows an image of me in a plaid shirt with camels. "Please, ma'am, shoes are not allowed in the studio," one says, respectful in a half bow. I sit barefoot on a stool for the interview, the bright-pink silk dupatta slipping from my neck. In English, we discuss the fate of camels and the power of their milk. The show will air once it's been translated into Hindi.

A reporter drives me to Samode Haveli, a palace in the Old City that's become a hotel, the fate of many Indian palaces whose owners need the money. Jaipur is called the Pink City for its softly salmon buildings, painted this color for a Victorian royal visit. I pass a pink palace with jalousies, honeycomb windows that once let concealed women look out. Painted white lines arch above them like eyebrows. After checking in, I wander to the Samode's plush library, furnished with red velvet sofas and chandeliers. Classic Indian patterns in silver, blue, red, and yellow glow on the ceilings and walls. A corner nook beckons, decorated in delft blue and white. Another niche glimmers forest green under an emerald lamp. The fan spins lazily above, these days turned by electricity instead of a servant. It would be easy for a visitor to play maharani here, secluded from the outside world. But the inevitable progress that toppled the Raj is the reason I'm here today.

The camel's economic value is falling faster than that of a stereo in the digital age. It's been designated the state animal of Rajasthan, which sounds protective. But this law means it's forbidden to take camels out of state. People who once used them for transportation or on farms now choose trucks and tractors, making camels obsolete. Muslim markets hanker for camel meat, especially for Eid sacrifices and Ramadan feasts, but animal slaughter is taboo to many Hindus, and eating meat is becoming more controversial. The only good camel markets are now outside the state and in foreign countries, but smuggling them is risky work, as the routes are increasingly policed. Even legitimate camel owners are being accused of smuggling. Religious tensions have resulted in their being beaten by crowds for "being Muslim," even if they aren't. Other restrictions have hampered some city camel rides for tourists. Camel use is dropping under its own protective burden.

Some camel owners are pinning their last hopes on milk, now sort of legally for sale after years of work by local activists. Perhaps this was helped (who knows?) by an article I wrote for openDemocracy about camel herders and their advocates. Few Indians drink camel milk apart from castes like the Raika, a group of herders or pastoralists who are said to shun outside contact. Today's paper carried a story with a photo of my son and me smiling under the curvy Hindi script. Tomorrow I'll give a presentation on camel milk's benefits, organized by a local newspaper for an audience of reporters, academics, and whoever else shows up.

In the morning my taxi swims slowly through the Old City traffic among a school of motorbikes, auto-rickshaws, horses, and bowed men pushing loaded carts. At an upscale vegetarian restaurant I reunite with Dr. Ilse Köhler-Rollefson, a German vet who settled in India after falling in love with camels — and with her local camel expert and guide, now her partner, Hanwant Singh Rathore. She's been advocating for Raika people and their camels for twenty years, with mixed results. Winning over the Raika took time (they love her), as did convincing them to sell their milk. She has also struggled with food authorities, grazing issues, and herd management. Now she's invited me here to support her mission. I'll go to her camel festival, too — and spend time with the herders, visit a special-needs school, and speak at a disability conference. ("You'll help the kids, Mom, won't you?" Jonah had solemnly asked. My heart melted with pride in him.)

After pizza and samosas, we arrive at the stunning castle housing the Rajasthan Patrika media group, the publisher of India's eighth-largest newspaper. In a pale-green conference room, a tall man gently smiles and extends his hand. "I am Dr. Agrawal. I work at the National Research Centre on Camel in Bikaner."

I'm astonished. "Of course, I know your work, with diabetes and the Raika!"

He hands me a set of his papers. "Please enjoy."

For years I have read the words attributed, in the dry bylines of science, to R. P. Agrawal. His fascinating references to the Raika were another reason for me to investigate the mysteries of camel milk. Diabetes, now a major health concern in India, is virtually unknown among Raika camel-herding communities. This can be attributed partly to their active lifestyle, but the consumption of camel milk may play a role. Dr. Agrawal, who studies the Raika, thinks that the insulin found in camel milk might be better absorbed into the bloodstream than that of other milks and thus help regulate blood sugar more effectively. He's shown that camel milk improves pancreatic function. Most significantly, his study showed that camel milk reduced blood sugar levels in twelve patients with type 1 diabetes, three of whom were able to discontinue taking insulin. He's presenting today too.

The other panelists include Ilse and Hanwant, who help run a Raika camel dairy, and the minister of animal husbandry. In keeping with ministerial tradition, he has not yet arrived. We walk to a large, packed room and sit before a gorgeous blue banner of camels. Men start giving speeches, even though they aren't panelists. Their words sound strong, almost harsh to my ear, and I don't understand a thing, but everyone's mood is positive.

Dr. Agrawal gives his crisply scientific talk in English mixed with Hindi. Ilse, tall with a crop of wavy red hair, makes an impassioned plea in Hindi for the camels. *Is she crying?* I wonder. But no. Maybe it's just years of frustration combined with the language. Such institutional head-banging would fell lesser folks.

More people arrive and start lining the walls. "People saw the article in the *Patrika*, and they are coming. It was supposed to be a small event," Ilse whispers. A dad waves his small son's wrist at me. The boy has Down syndrome (it's estimated that 20 to 40 percent of Down syndrome patients have autism). Two men in red, green, and yellow turbans and white tunics sit in the back, clearly different in occupation from the others wearing saris and business attire. Loudspeakers are set up for people listening outside.

Now I'm handed the microphone. "How many people have family members with autism?" I ask. Many hands go up. "How many are professionals helping autism?" More hands, perhaps half the audience. There are an estimated ten million people with autism in India, and that's probably an undercount, as in most countries — including the United States. "Autism families are the same all over the world. I consider you my brothers and sisters, so welcome," I say.

I go through my son's story and discuss others' anecdotes and scientific studies. I explain why camel milk might help with autism, who might benefit, and the eternal question, how much to give a child (or adult). The minister arrives, in a khaki uniform and rainbow-swirl turban, but people wait for me to resume. I tell them to think like a scientist, to change only one thing in a child's diet or routine at a time, and I explain how to observe and record data. I caution them on milk safety and advise them to eliminate cow milk first (saying this quickly in the land of sacred cows). I mention that yeast, a fungus, can cause behavioral and physical symptoms, and recommend cutting down on yeast-nourishing carbohydrates such as bread and rice, and sweets like gulab jamun, a fried milk dumpling soaked in syrup. When I finish, the room erupts with comments and questions.

"We have to wait until the panel is over!" says Ilse. As the minister speaks, the two turbaned men rise and question him sharply. They are camel herders. The minister lobs back his own replies, waving his arms. "Time for questions," says Ilse.

The pent-up wave breaks. "Madam, I am a colonel of the army, and please tell me, my grandchild has autism, how much can I give her?" This man shares details of the therapies the family has tried, just like every autism family in the world, and presses a letter with the girl's history into my hand. People reach for the microphone. "Hello, please, hello, my son has autism, and what kind of diet did you say?" "Hello, please, Madam — " Six people talk while dozens more wave their hands and crowd the table. A man holds a child out to me. "I have to ask you, how much my son needs, his doctor says he have autism, what do I do?" A commanding woman in a red-gold sari takes the mic. "Hal-lo, hal-lo!!" she shouts. "I want to ask you a question, I work with the association and my child has autism — " It's chaos.

"I promise I will stay until I can get to everyone." I keep answering, but as people line up three deep, a moderator dismisses the crowd. "Come to the back," says one host.

"But I said I would help them," I say, appalled at the idea of letting them down.

"Don't worry, they can email you. We had planned a reception for you with journalists now, but so many people came we canceled it. But can you please talk to them?"

After interviews at a patio picnic table, I'm taken to the great medieval-looking lair of the publisher. He nods kindly.

"We like to help the people," he says. He gives me a book he's written, with a pale-pink lotus on the cover. Then I'm outside the palace, my head still full of voices. The sun is warm and low in the sky, and the quiet makes me wonder if I made it all up.

Late that night, the phone rings in my hotel room. "Madam, can you please come to the lobby? You have a visitor."

"Who is it?"

"Someone from the police." The police? This can't be good.

I look at Tony. "It's the police. What should I do?"

He looks back at me, equally at a loss. "I don't know."

"I guess I can't say no. It's not like they have to get a warrant. If they want me, they can get me," I say.

"Do you know what they want?" I ask the clerk on the phone.

"He says he wants to talk to you. Will you come down?"

I take a deep breath. "Okay."

I look big-eyed at my husband. "Will you come with me?" I don't want to think this, but it might be the last time he sees me for a while. I've done nothing wrong, but in a foreign country, you never know.

Downstairs in the small reception area, a man is waiting. "Ma'am, you are Christina Adam?"

I gulp. Being close to law enforcement officials makes you feel guilty even if you aren't. "Yes. Did I do anything wrong?"

He smiles a bit. "Someone wants to talk to you." He gestures to the phone in the desk clerk's hand. "Hello?"

A deep voice speaks. He's a high-level official. "I saw the article in the paper. I have a child with autism," he starts. I sigh with relief. "Can you meet with me?" he asks.

"I'm leaving tomorrow at noon, but if you can come here, I will be glad to talk."

"Okay, I will be there."

Tony punches my arm teasingly. "See? Nothing to worry about!"

The next day, a smooth-haired young woman waits alone in the grassy courtyard, framed by the palace's pillars. "My husband was called to the High Court, but I wanted to meet you. Is that okay?"

Under the arches of the pale-green dining room, she tells me about her child. I lead her through the steps of early autism intervention, knowing the gentleness a parent needs to help a child through this diagnosis. In her face I see fear, unspilled tears, and an iron resolve. I don't know if I'll hear from her again. But it doesn't matter. We will always be a memory to one another.

Now, I'm heading into the desert, to meet the camel herders of Rajasthan and learn about the forces that drive them.

29 AN OLD CAMEL CASTE IN THE NEW INDIA

"Big problem. Camels are day by day less."
— Netha Raika

A scarlet-draped cart jangles down the sandy back road on the way to the famed Pushkar Camel Fair, its big back tires rolling through the ruts. A family sits cross-legged on flowered cushions inside. A camel trots between the cart's curved wooden shafts, ankle bells tinkling, caramel body and legs stretching over the dust. Stately yet utterly unconcerned, it wears a colorful, tasseled mesh cloth on its hump, and red and green garlands are wound around its neck. Fluffy balls above a yellow halter adorn its nose, which is pierced with wood. The charcoal-colored circular splotches on its cheek and the dotted willow tree on its haunch are the marks of its owner. The sandaled driver holds the thin reins casually as my taxi rolls right up behind him with a high-pitched beep, confirming that camels don't easily startle. We flash past two, three, four decorated carts and a camel wearing beads around its neck. The trees give way to power lines and scraggly plants, then I see tents on a rise in the distance.

I've been calling Netha Raika, a Facebook friend who can barely write English but has made plain his distress about the fading of Raika camel culture. We can't figure out where to meet because I don't know the landmarks. The driver takes my phone. They shout in a language I can't identify: Hindi? Marwadi? I think they're arguing, but no, it's just the way they speak. "You wait tea stand, he will come," the driver says. Once I exit, with Tony soldierlike at my back, the peddlers descend. "Necklace, bracelet, very good quality, you look, madam," they chant, lifting necklaces to my eyes. "No, thank you, maybe later," I reply, and scan the fluttering tents, with their prayer flags, rugs, potato chip packets, and statues. Wrong tea stand. There are no herders here.

Three men in saffron, orange, and green turbans approach, beating a drum. A live gunmetal serpent is draping the neck of a handsome man in jeans, whose black hair curls to the collar of his tunic. A shirtless little boy hovers nearby, his face painted white with a black mustache. His peach turban is topped by a black cobra head. A smaller boy in vivid pink asks for money in his husky baby voice. "This is my family," says the snake-wearing man. The snake's tail quivers in midair. "Probably defanged," says an onlooker, but Tony drops money into the boy's basket.

Finally I see Netha, as slim and intense as he appears online. "Hello, Adams-ji," he says with a shy smile.

I first glimpsed Netha in photos showing him crouched in his living room, offering handmade camel decorations for sale. I saw pictures of his newborn girl, but no wife (local customs dictate not to ask about wives). He messaged me in a form of jumbled English I named Googlish (he probably used Google Translate). Inspired by his lonely devotion to camels, I wrote an article about his dying culture. Now, in the midday Pushkar sun, I stretch my hand out and take his.

"You please follow with me," he says, smiling. He's wearing slightly rumpled Western slacks and a polo shirt — no traditional white tunic today.

We walk up the hot asphalt road toward an open-air tea stall. Half a dozen Raika men sit on a camel-hair rug below it. Their turbans are red, yellow, or dazzling multicolor with white dots.

The men are surrounded by camels — camels with lean legs and toothy "smiles," camels with curly hair and soft eyes, humps shaved in tufts and blackened with dye, white scars in arcs from ears to cheek, ears like a Viking's horns. Their necks are wrapped in white shells, their coats branded with button-like circles.

Two camels stand like bookends, inches apart. Others saunter easily among the herd, stepping nonchalantly between reclining humps and splayed legs. Some lie with their heads on the ground, necks flat as they stare from the dirt. An older camel rests on its wrinkled back knees, forelegs stretched on a carpet like a dog.

"Is there a tent?"

"We no using tents," Netha says. The starry sky is their roof. They've walked three nights to get here, sleeping by day.

"Is everyone here Raika?"

"Ninety percent Raika peoples selling camel here, 10 percent other peoples." A Raika man flashes behind Netha, his stick upraised as he drives a jingling camel toward the road. "Raika community doing camel breeding — no other peoples interested. Long, long time to bring this work."

The Raika have a mission: taking care of camels. According to their creation story, Parvati, the goddess consort of Lord Shiva, made a strange five-legged animal from clay and asked Shiva to give it life. He declined, thinking the beast could not thrive, but finally gave in. When it couldn't walk well, "Shiva his hands to down one leg," says Netha, showing how he shaped the leftover limb into a hump. So great were the camel's needs that Parvati sought a caregiver for it. So Shiva made the first Raika from the dust, says Netha. He learned this story from the older Raika of his community. They have another deity, Pabuji, "our simple god," says Netha. "When our camel sick, we pray to Pabuji, then good health."

For the clannish Raika, it is still somewhat taboo to sell camel milk to anyone. A few years ago a sales scheme was proposed, but according to rumor it was sabotaged by dipping camels' unclean tails in the milk, thus threatening the health of would-be consumers. There's still no camel dairy industry in India, other than Ilse's nascent operation and a few small providers. I've assumed that most Raika would be willing to sell milk if it kept their camels alive. But you can't assume anything about India, especially if you aren't Indian. It's a market awash in intercultural failures. Now that I'm about to meet them, it hits me that I don't know if they will sell it now.

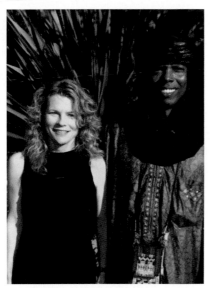

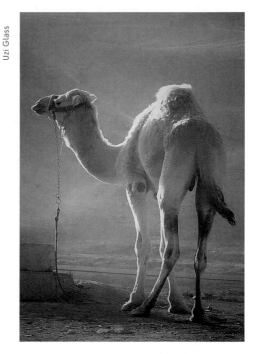

Christina meeting Elhadji Koumama during his visit to Orange County, California. His nomadic Tuareg family has made silver jewelry for twenty-five generations.

A white camel outside Jericho in the West Bank.

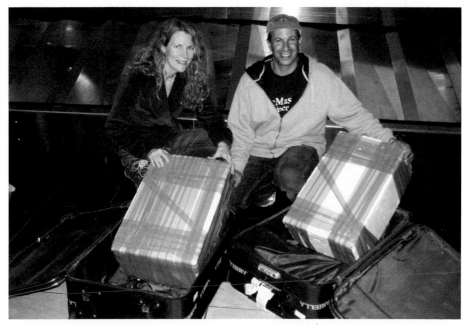

Christina receiving a shipment of Bedouin camel milk at an airport with the help of Gil Riegler.

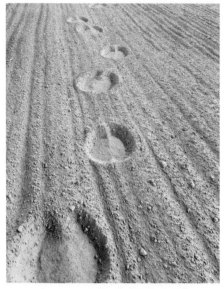

Camel footprints in the sand. Their soft padded feet give them stability on shifting sands like those of the ancient Silk Road trading routes.

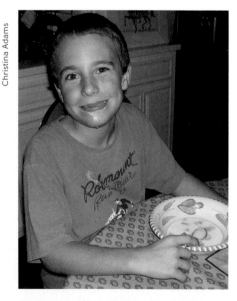

Big Iwan, a famous Bactrian camel in Belgium, gives his owner, Karin den Hartog-Peute, a ride.

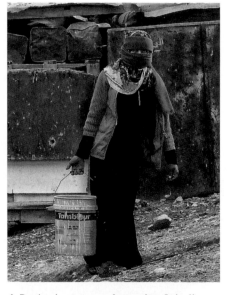

A Bedouin woman from the Jahalin tribe carries a bucket in the Judean Desert. Her group lives in tents in the West Bank.

Jonah drinking camel milk for the first time.

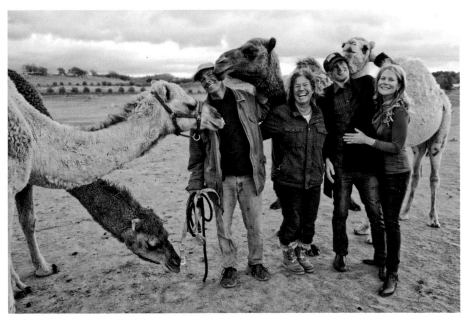

Gil and Nancy Riegler share their camels with Tony and Christina Adams, Oasis Camel Dairy, Ramona, California.

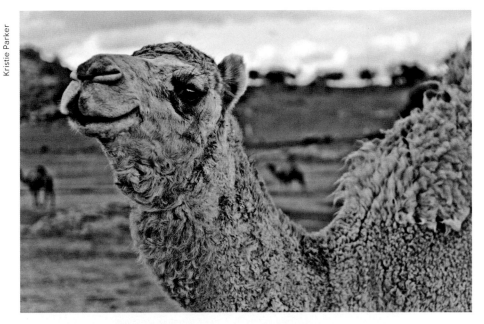

A happy camel at Oasis Camel Dairy, Ramona, California.

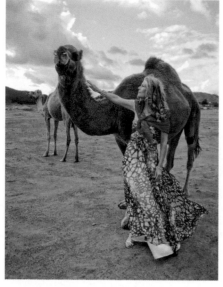

Kristie Parker

Christina connects with Cleopatra at Oasis Camel Dairy, Ramona, California.

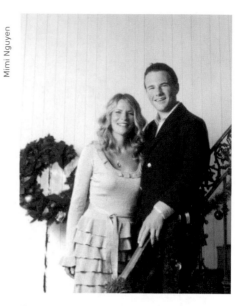

Mimi Nguyen

Christina and Jonah at home.

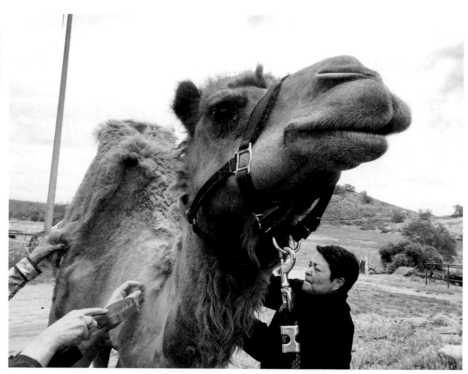

Christina Adams

American women learn camel grooming at popular hands-on clinics at Oasis Camel Dairy, Ramona, California.

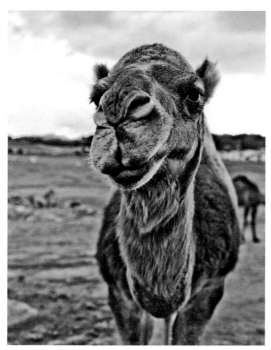

Grumpy? Skeptical? A camel
eyes onlookers at Oasis Camel
Dairy, Ramona, California.

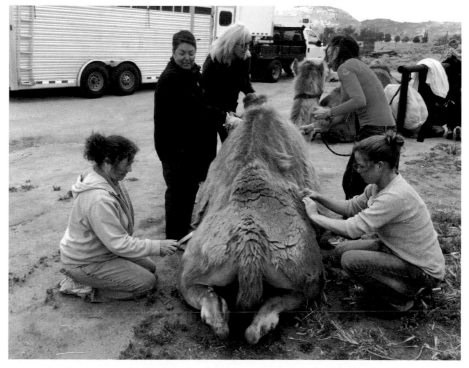

Nancy Riegler (*left*) teaches camel grooming at Oasis Camel Dairy,
Ramona, California.

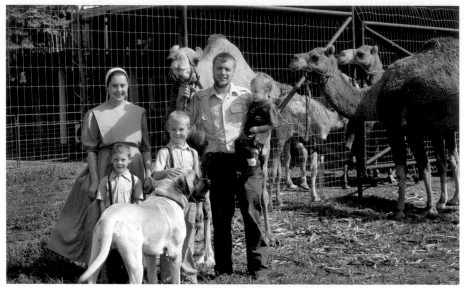

Mennonite camel farmers Savannah and Marlin Troyer with three of their sons —
from left to right, Tristan, Ray, and Bradley — at their Michigan camel farm.

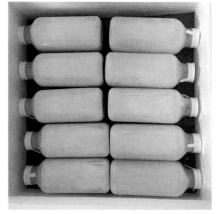

Bottles of frozen American camel milk.

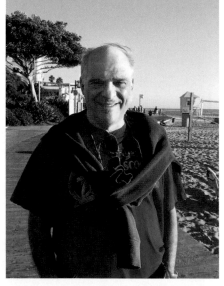

Dr. Amnon Gonenne visits Christina in
Orange County, California. Their initial
connection led to her son's successful
treatment with camel milk.

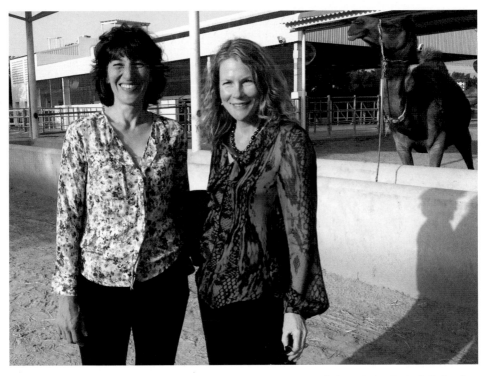

Camel veterinarian Dr. Jutka Juhász and Christina at Camelicious farm, Dubai, United Arab Emirates. Dr. Jutka is widely known for her work with camels and is popular with her staff.

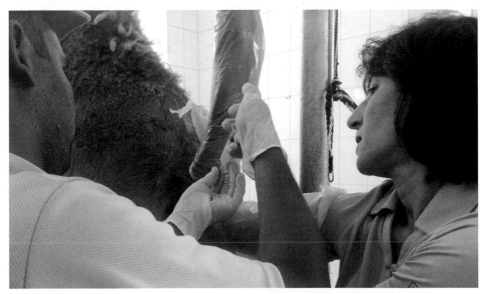

Dr. Jutka Juhász, wearing a full-length glove, and her helper transfer a camel embryo into a female camel at Camelicious, Dubai.

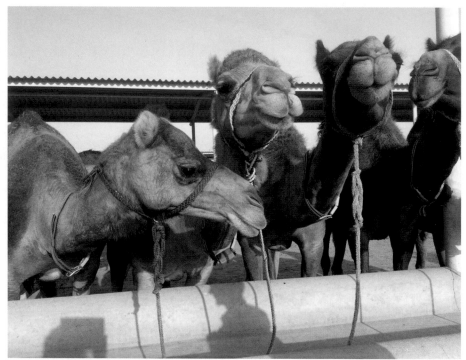

Retired camels greet visitors to Camelicious, Dubai.

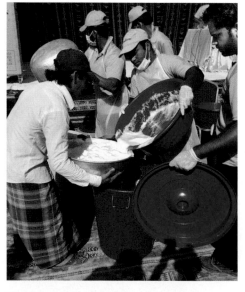

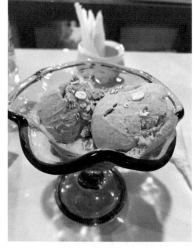

Camel milk ice cream at the Arabian Tea House, Dubai.

The Camelicious team competing in the camel-milking contest at a heritage festival, Dubai.

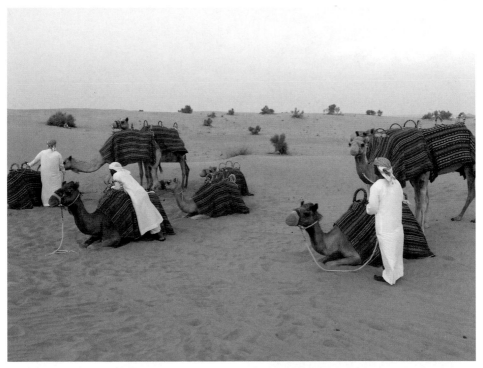

In the Dubai Desert Conservation Reserve, which constitutes nearly 5 percent of the area of Dubai, tour guides lead camel treks through the desert.

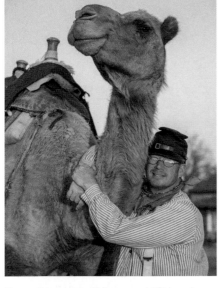

Doug Baum and his camel Richard at Fort Chadbourne, Texas, where he reenacts the historic US Army camel experiment of the 1850s.

Bhanwarlal Raika milks a camel into a pot in Sadri, India. The herders will sip milk and a traditional mild narcotic tea after the morning milking.

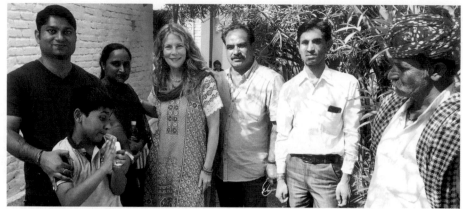

From left to right: A family with an autistic child, Christina, Hanwant Singh Rathore of Camel Charisma, and others, Sadri, India.

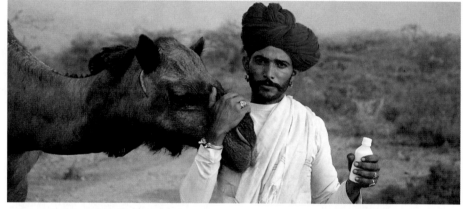

Herder Bhanwarlal Raika holds a bottle of camel milk near Sadri, India.

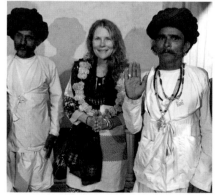

Christina being honored at a Raika community temple near Ranakpur, India.

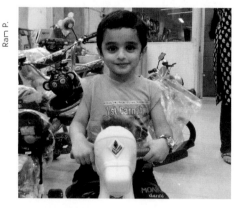

A boy in Chennai, India, whose father says 85 percent of his autism symptoms were addressed by camel milk from Dr. Ilse Köhler-Rollefson's camel dairy.

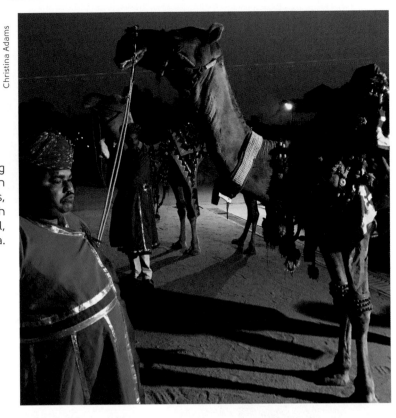

An evening
procession
with camels,
Rambagh
Palace Hotel,
Jaipur, India.

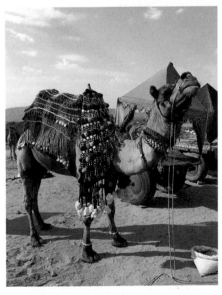

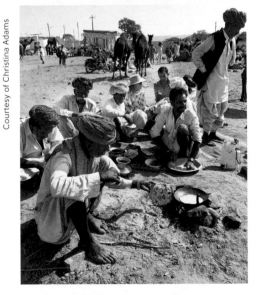

A colorful decorated camel and cart,
Pushkar Camel Fair, Pushkar, India. The
decline in camel-based transportation
has lessened demand for the animals.

Christina meeting Raika herders at the
Pushkar Camel Fair with Netha Raika
(*in blue shirt*).

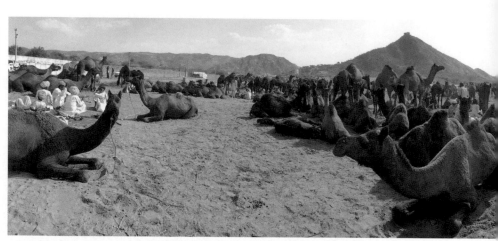

An increasingly bare campground at the Pushkar Camel Fair, Pushkar, India, reflects the desolation felt by Raika herders due to falling camel prices.

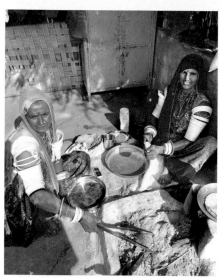

Sukhi Devi (*left*) and Samu Devi cooking millet roti near Pichiyak, India. Fresh sheep milk is kept in the cabinet.

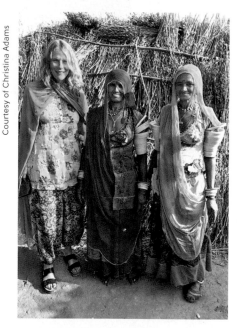

Christina and Raika sheepherders Samu Devi (*left*) and Sukhi Devi outside their field shelter, called a *jhupdi*, near Pichiyak, India.

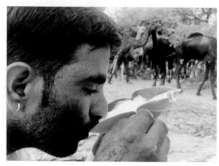

Magan Raika drinking camel milk from a traditional aak-leaf cup in Sadri, India. Some say the leaf is poisonous, but others say a drop of the sap has medicinal benefits.

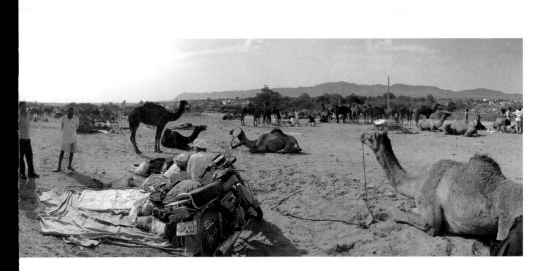

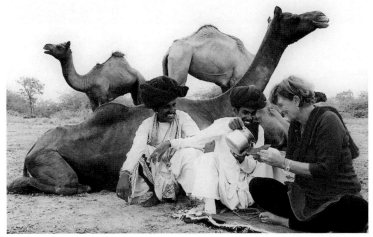

Two Raika herders (*center*, Madaram Raika) and Dr. Ilse Köhler-Rollefson enjoy local camel milk served in the traditional aak-leaf cup near Sadri, India.

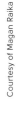

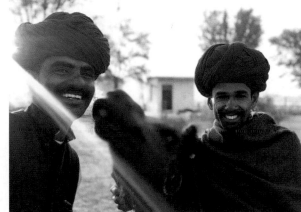

Magan Raika and Madaram Raika having fun with a camel in Sadri, India.

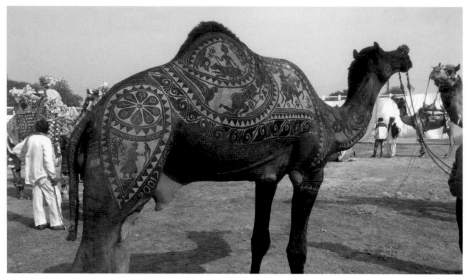

A decorated camel at the Bikaner Camel Festival, Bikaner, India. Scissors are used to cut designs into the camel's hair, and dye is used to darken the head, legs, and tip of the hump.

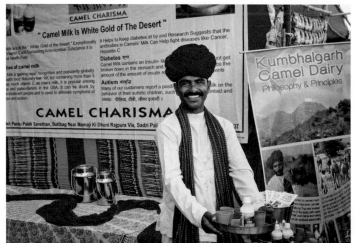

Magan Raika raises awareness of camel milk at the Pushkar Camel Fair, Pushkar, India. Selling milk offers one way to save camels and preserve traditional herder lifestyles.

Camel herder Magan Raika with his friend near Sadri, India. According to the Raika people's origin story, they were created by Lord Shiva to take care of camels.

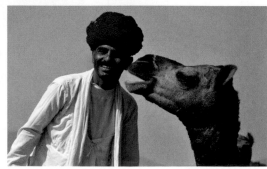

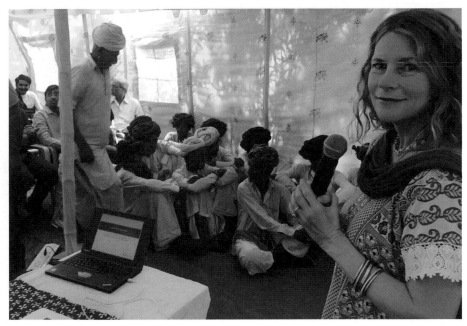

Raika camel herders at Christina's lecture at the Marwar Camel Festival in Sadri, India.

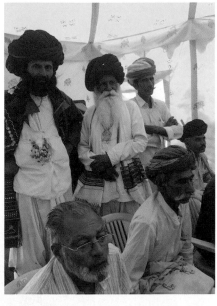

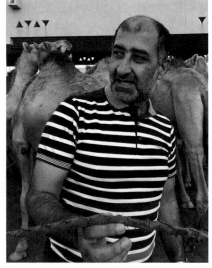

Raika, Maru, and Rajput men attend Christina's lecture in Sadri, India.

The Pakistani veterinarian and plant expert Abdul Raziq Kakar shares his traditional knowledge at the Al Ain camel souk (market), Abu Dhabi, United Arab Emirates.

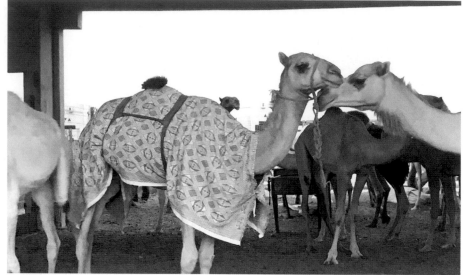

A black-tufted racing camel communicates with another, Al Ain camel souk (market), Abu Dhabi.

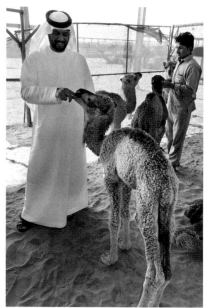

Mubarak, the farm manager, and a farmworker with baby camels at Al Ain Farms, Abu Dhabi.

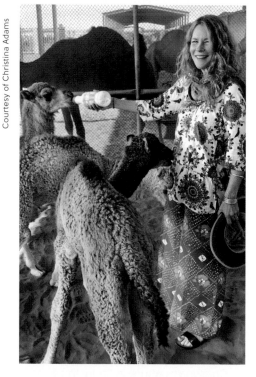

Christina with baby camels at Al Ain Farms. Babies are kept close to their mothers after birth.

Dirt grinds under my feet as we approach. Netha points to the rug. "Should we take shoes off?" I ask.

"Shoes is okay now, Adams-ji, you no worry."

I sit. The curled brown edge of the rug is barely distinguishable from the dirt. Maroon and mustard blankets are heaped on a large white sugar sack. Like their camels, the men sit facing mostly in the same direction, their backs turned as Netha speaks to them in what he says is Marwadi. A small-humped *unt* (camel, also spelled *oont*) arches its head over us. The rest of the herd stands or lounges nearby, their long necks looped with fraying red cord.

Two men turn and nod. Netha speaks to a shoeless man with no turban.

"You say you want Raika meal, this is Raika food."

One of the ways Indian men court your friendship online (or sometimes more, but thankfully not in Netha's case) is by sending photos of their food: stainless-steel *thali*s (platters) with bowls of raita (yogurt and cucumber sauce) and algae-green mint chutney, charred round roti (bread) with stewed dal (lentils) of yellow and black, thick brown spoonfuls of chana masala (chickpeas in gravy). I once casually told Netha I wanted some if I ever made it back to Rajasthan. Now he's offering what once seemed an impossible meal.

The barefoot cook kneads dough in a tin pan. Under his small rolling pin, a perfect six-inch circle emerges, which he cooks on an iron skillet over a small fire. Netha places the chewy, black-blistered roti in my hand. I tear off pieces as I sip hot tea with milk (cow, not camel). Bits of dirt crunch in my teeth. The men, their white sleeves pulled back or rolled to show watches, silver bracelets, or red strings, take roti too.

It's amazing to be here. But my joy is tempered with a sudden realization. Three to four years ago, ten thousand camels filled this brown valley. Today, "official count is 2,800," says Netha. The bare ground tells the desolate story. "Five years ago, this ground only camels, camels. No space. But you can see now very space, camels are only little. Big problem," says Netha mournfully. "Camels are day by day less."

"These camels are hobbled," I say, looking at the camels surrounding us. A thin rope lifts one foreleg of each camel and ties it up behind the bent knee, keeping the foot off the ground. The camels walk in a three-legged teeter. It doesn't appear to bother them.

"So they no go to other place," he explains.

Nearby is an unt the color of blackened toast. Its lower lip hangs unnaturally, exposing the skewed teeth in a macabre grin. "Oh, what happened to it, Netha?"

"Owner say it was caught on a pen," he says. "No have money to fix."

Netha tells the men I am a camel milk promoter (not exactly, but oh well) and takes out the newspaper article from Jaipur. They pass it around, but I know most cannot read. "Do you have camels' medicine, they asking?" says Netha. "Mange big problem now." No, I don't.

Netha explains to them that I am going to Sadri next, where Ilse is helping a different group of Raika to sell camel milk. A man in a pale-yellow turban gestures to the groans and mumbling of the camels.

"Sadri is very big distance from here," Netha translates. It's at least a five-hour drive, but for nomads with limited access to cars it might as well be a thousand miles, especially with camels. They have no way to transport milk that far.

"Tell them I will talk about ways to keep milk cold and move it in Sadri." Netha won't be there either — it's too far for him — but he can share my lecture in the Raika oral tradition. "By the way, how has your English gotten so good so fast?" He smiles shyly and just dips his head. I wish I could speak his language at all.

Two Raika walk up, one man's arm slung over the other's shoulder. Netha shows them the newspaper, but they seem frustrated. "No good," one says in Marwadi.

Netha tells them over 150 people came to the meeting in Jaipur hoping to get camel milk.

"It says please buy, please buy, but we are in the forest, so how can we be contacted?" the man exclaims to Netha. "One day here, two days there, very hard life." He blames a common culprit. "Government," he says sardonically, flipping his fingers in dismissal. He smiles as they leave.

"Why are people asking for government help here? They can legally sell camel milk now," I say, although I know some bureaucratic hurdles remain. "I guess it's the camel sales restrictions." After all, these guys are breeders and traders, not dairy folks.

"Government policy is no good," Netha says. The Raika's grazing access has been progressively reduced, resulting in poor nutrition and increased disease for the camels. Additionally, no one knows what to do with male camels if they can't be sold outside Rajasthan. "Second problem, young generation necessary interest. If not, automatically camel count grow thin." I realize Netha is the only one of his age here. He has stayed despite having enough education to find a place elsewhere. He wants to help his culture, but he must be a little camel crazy too.

A stocky Raika man comes over, face stern under his slanted red turban. He has a black handlebar mustache and a silver bracelet and ring on each hand. Two others join him. Netha speaks, but the man doesn't smile, just stares past my shoulder. He lights a small green cigarette, blowing smoke from his nose like a bull. "What's that?" I ask.

He holds out a rolled leaf tied with a tiny red string. I take the little scroll between two fingers, decide to go for it, and coolly blow twin streams from my nostrils.

"Awwww!" they exclaim and laugh. A smile crosses his face. "Very good, you like *beedi*," Netha translates for him. I don't smoke, but this is a pretty flavorful little cigarette.

"I like your bracelet," I say.

"Hmm," the man says. When he speaks, Netha looks uneasy and shakes his head.

"What is it?"

"He says, sister, he will trade his ring for that one."

He's pointing to the ruby solitaire on my hand. The pigeon's-blood stone isn't great quality, but it's set in my original engagement ring. The man holds out a pewter-colored ring bearing an oval shield with a camel.

"You no have to," Netha says nervously.

Should I do it? The man watches me weigh the idea. I think, *Maybe he can throw in a camel.* Tony stands innocently a few feet behind me. I shake my head.

"Tony-ji probably no like it," Netha says, proving that he and Tony are getting along well.

"I can't, my husband gave it to me," I concede. Tony steps over. "Do you like his ring? I can trade yours for it," I say, laughing. He looks at the little camel ring.

"Nice. But I don't think so."

"I really appreciate it, but this is my wedding jewelry," I tell him through Netha, hoping this reason has cross-cultural weight.

"Tell Hollywood your husband won't allow it," says Tony. I see what he's alluding to: there is something theatrical and dashing about the guy. Hollywood shrugs ruefully, still trying to do the deal with his eyes. I shake my head and smile. But I wish I could...

"Photo?" Hollywood and I stand together, his delicious beedi in my fingers, his face forbidding over folded arms.

"Now camels going to forest," Netha says. His people take them for an afternoon graze before returning for the evening bed-down. The camels lift themselves from the ground and amble down the asphalt in a glorious parade. Tourists and photographers scramble alongside for pictures. The camels need almost no prodding. They know what to do. There's no flinching or shying like with horses, no bucking or twisting heads. There's a slowness to their limbs even when they run. Perhaps this is why I find them so calming.

Yards away, a large stone trough serves as both human bathtub and camel watering hole. A young man removes his clothes and sluices water over his chest and tight black underwear. The camels drink, dipping their heads, then looking around in their peculiar fixed way. They don't crowd each other or fight. The herders in multicolored turbans are Maru Raika, like Netha. Red may or may not signify Godwari Raika. Each group lives in a different region. Although I know that Raika women manage camels, goats, and sheep, I see no herder women here.

There are a few foreign men and women, who mostly look like me. They don't sit or speak to anyone. They walk by, gaze at us, and leave.

If you are intimidated by groups of men in turbans, you will not come to this section of the fair. If you are afraid of large animals, you will stick to the road. If you want necklaces or statues, you will leave for town. And you will miss the heart of this culture, unaware of its hidden marvels.

The next day, we reconvene on the rug with two bags of barbecue-flavor potato chips. I bought them as a snack for the herders, but the two men I hand them to eat them all. I have the roti and tea.

Everyone's still hoping to sell some camels, but time is running out. "The government only allow so many days for the fair as the holy festival starts soon," Netha explains. Camel brokers have been arriving not just from Rajasthan but from Uttar Pradesh, Delhi, and Hyderabad.

"But you aren't supposed to move them outside of Rajasthan now," I say.

Netha dips his head. "Out of state peoples are coming, but only little peoples now." The law seems to be having an effect, but traffic continues — camel smugglers using trucks are sometimes caught by the army.

Beside the rug squats Danaram-ji, an elderly Raika in a canary-yellow turban, his bunched white pantaloons brushing the pebbled dirt. An owner of twenty-four camels, he brought four males here to sell. Under his brushy white mustache he smiles cheerfully, holding a rolled roti in one hand, a curved stick in the other.

"He is old now, two years no doing business," says Netha. "But he is young," he adds, pointing at his brother-in-law's "small brother," Babulal-ji. "He no income or resource than selling camels. He only now ten camels." This is dire, because the Pushkar Fair may bring in most of the year's income.

Babulal-ji sits across from me, wearing a gold floral earring and a white snap-front shirt tagged Kohinoor, for the largest Indian diamond ever found. He's sitting cross-legged in the same sort of pants as Danaram-ji. Most camel herders are over fifty years old, but only the barest wisps of gray touch his thatched haircut. Yet his face is pained. He waggles his head from side to side, speaking in a low, husky voice.

"He's here for four days, with three camels to sell," Netha translates, "but no selling camels. He is asking fifteen thousand rupees [around US $220], but broker only offered five to eight thousand rupees. Then he agreed to twelve thousand, but broker is only offer eight thousand." And the broker has not yet returned with the money.

"That's a low price!" I say. "Bad business model."

"So he is now angry, waiting here for four days."

"If he no selling camels, what will he do?" I ask, unconsciously adopting his phrasing.

"He will try to sell them another fair."

"How does he keep feeding them?"

"He feeding only on local food and grass," Netha says.

"He have any children interested in camel business?"

"Young people like technology. Camel business no technology. Cow business very technical now, and many peoples are dairy farming. But camels no are dairy farming."

"When he can't keep them anymore, will he sell at the low price?" I ask.

"If no selling, then he will no doing camel business."

"Oh, he'll quit?"

"He have new business in sheep. One sheep selling four to five thousand rupees." Their meat is sold to Muslims, their manure as fertilizer. "One sheep takes six months to breed, so two times a year for sheep. Camels are two years to breed, then only have one animal," says Netha. "Camel is very loss business."

As the camels burble and groan, lazing peacefully among their caregivers, it's clear no camel rescuer is coming. No government officials are here, no international aid representatives are taking notes.

"Government say, why you want camel, you no need."

"Young people no want camels."

This is what the Raika have been told.

These men do a good job of hiding their desperation. But how does it feel when your leaders and your own children scoff at your hallowed way of life?

But Netha has news. "Sister, I am going to open a camel center and dairy." He will operate it for tourists, teach people about camels, and maybe, just maybe, keep his people linked to camels. "I am working for camel conservation. This is my duty."

"Great, Netha," I say slowly. "How will you afford it?"

"My family help me to buy land."

It seems unnatural and ironic that nomads must buy land in order to share their culture with tourists. But unfair or not, maybe paying for land offers a way for Netha to save shreds of the camel lifestyle.

"I wish you the best, Netha. If I can do anything to help, let me know."

"Thank you, sister." We stand quietly as camel grunts and moans float through the dusty valley.

Netha is a brave person. Perhaps he's dreaming. The dirt around us is a sea of despair, yet he persists. Maybe camel is not very loss business. His courage enriches us all.

30 HELP IN SUFFERING

"We smell and say, this is disease."
— OWNER OF ONE HUNDRED CAMELS

The Pushkar Fair also has a tent-and-wagon section, which is located across from the Raika camp. I wander over, floating among the few tourists in this stretch of powdery dirt, and find the performing camels. Gorgeous in handcrafted decorations, they're ringed, belled, dyed, and decked out. Elaborate patterns of birds, leaves, and flowers are clipped with scissors into their coats. A starred cheek lies beneath dyed black hair that's sculpted to resemble a snood. Black kohl outlines their eyes, Bollywood style. Floral collars adorn pale necks. One camel tilts its flower-tipped nose and emits a bored moo. Well-nourished and content, they watch the scene inscrutably.

A man in a sleeveless shirt and rubber thongs unties a tall, tawny camel, its huge liquid eye dark as a date. "Cloud," says the Indian script on its shoulder. A flowerpot design grows a stem up the belly to a black-dyed ruff of hump hair. The camel's legs are shorn down to the upper thighs, leaving furry showgirl stockings. "B.S.," its owner's initials, slant down the neck. A flowery mandala on the rump flows into a comet trailing a phone number down the leg. The owner steps back and motions to the camel. It pounds the dirt with its front feet, "dancing," as its owner says with a proud grin. As the camel rhythmically stomps, as if doing laundry in a tub, the man snaps a small strap once against its neck.

I look around. There have been minor animal rights protests against camel riding in a few cities. I've seen videos of camels at festivals leaping over people and rearing high on their hind legs while wearing finery, but one expert says no camels have been injured by such activities in his camel-rich area. At any rate, I spot none of these displays or protesters today. Owners of highly trained camels and horses, generally very poor people who make their living this way, are respected here.

A camel cart draws close, and some tourists gather round it. The pale-beige, jingle-belled camel pulling it is mottled with black patches. "What's that?" asks one woman. "Mange," says an onlooker. This common parasitic skin infection is treated with folk remedies (which are somewhat effective) or donated medicine. But with Raika resources stretched this year and no donors, there's no easy solution. The lack of good grazing land has weakened the camels and made them more prone to infections. Mange can irritate and even kill a camel, but the treatment is fairly cheap, in mainstream medicine terms if not Raika dollars. I spot empty bottles of ceftriaxone, an antibiotic, and meloxicam, an anti-inflammatory, in the dirt. At least the camels are getting some medical treatment.

The tourists spy another camel. "Do they spit?" asks a languid older blonde.

A little shiver runs through their group. Thanks to Doug Baum, I know that's regurgitation, not spit, but still I am not worried. I've been told that if they toss their heads and start growling, it's best to move, but this one is doing fine.

"What about these things?" asks a woman, pointing to the wooden points protruding from a camel's pierced nose.

She's pointing to a nose peg. As her group discusses them, I recall that the pegs are used to control male camels. People have tried to dissuade the Raika from using them, but to no avail. But it's not just the Raika — some Australians reportedly use them for the country's many feral camels. Rutting bull camels are a fearsome sight in any country.

Without nose pegs, male camels can be very difficult for some people to handle, unless extensive training practices, pens, or restraints are implemented. In India, where camels are typically not contained by fences and barns, uncontrolled bulls have attacked people. Some handlers say the solution is castration, as many cameleers practice in the US (where nose pegs are not used), adding that males grow bigger, stronger, and less aggressive if "cut" at two to four years old. But castration has been another Raika no-no. Netha says it's against their religion as camel caregivers, although his people castrate male goats. Doing this to camels is simply not their way.

I leave the decorated camels behind to meet Netha at the Help in Suffering tent, a nonprofit organization that brings vets to attend to fair animals. The tent's yellow and red paisley backdrop advertises the "camel team," which makes free visits to sick camels in Jaipur and beyond. They even have a camel ambulance with a hydraulic lift. Bottles of medicine, hypodermic needles, and pamphlets sit on the counter.

"What's this?" I ask, holding a two-inch white plastic rod with a circular base and pointed tip.

"It's a nose peg," says Dr. Abhinav Swami, a young vet with wire glasses. "Wooden and metal ones can break off and cause damage, so if they're going to use nose pegs," he shrugs with resignation, "we at least replace them with plastic. It's clean and doesn't break as much." Here is another old-meets-new contradiction. The Raika prefer a type of wood that doesn't "make poison" in their camels, saying that the plastic pegs cause fever and nose problems.

"Oh," I say, remembering, "there's a camel with its lower lip hanging off. Can you fix it for free?"

"Yes, we can," he says gravely.

I tell Netha the good news. "Now the owner just has to bring it over," I say happily.

In the tent, a white-bearded man in a goldenrod turban sits with his walking stick, his hands circling as he talks. He's a former government official. "I have a hundred camels," Dr. Swami translates for him. "All my life, in the morning, we go take the soil with the urine in it. We smell and say, this is disease. And the sick camels are separated. We gave the feces of donkeys to treat all the diseases."

"Do you believe this?" another man asks the men.

"Donkey *milk* is good for disease," I chime in. I've never heard about feces.

The older man waves his arms, his voice soft but emphatic. "Bronchitis, allergies, bacterial and viral infection…camel milk is increasing the immunity, and then diseases very quickly recover. And sugar and mentally disorders," Netha translates. *Sugar* is a word used to describe diabetes, which I've heard even in Appalachia. "Mentally disorders" — well, I can guess what that means.

"I believe that too," I assure the elder. "My own son."

The talk turns to selling camel milk, with Netha translating the former official's remarks. "Some village have only ten to twenty camels, and village is a very big distance. Camel herders, other village, then other village," Netha relays, moving his hands to illustrate the distance between them, "collect it — very big problem. How do you collect camel milk, he is asking?"

"Dr. Ilse has gone to Africa to look at solar-powered chillers," I say. "They use the sun to chill the milk, solar power, no machine needed."

Netha explains it to the official. He asks through Netha, "Many people are asking raw camel milk?"

"Many are asking for raw now," I say. "But there needs to be a standard for testing the animals and milk. Vets like these need to test the camels. You don't want people drinking the milk if the camel has disease."

Outside the tent a heated discussion breaks out. An embarrassment has occurred. The owner of the camel with the torn lip feels some kind of shame. He came to get medicine for another camel, but he doesn't want to bring the injured one. But the vets talk with him. Then they turn their backs to allow for deliberation. He finally agrees.

He leads the dark-brown camel to the vet's area, accompanied by another Raika man. They cush the unwilling camel, their sinewy feet in leather slippers bracing against the rocky dirt. Its tail curls under like a monkey's. Dr. Swami and the owner are kneeling by the head when the camel changes its mind. Its back legs rise quickly, and its head rears high. "Hya, hya, hya!" says the owner as Dr. Swami leaps backward. The owner and a vet tech seize the camel's big head and push it down. The Raika helper and vet tech pull the rope tight. The tethered camel begins a hollow growl.

Dr. Swami pulls bits of flesh from the lower lip, dropping pieces into the dust. "The bone is in good shape, not cracked," he comments. The growl continues as three techs, two vets, the Raika men, and another man surround the camel, their hands pressing the head as in a benediction. More flesh is flicked from the latex glove. A tech swabs the wound. The camel continues to growl softly as it recovers. The Raika helper squats for a cigarette break, then rises and puts his slipper on the camel's neck to hold it down. An injection is over in seconds. The owner and his helper massage the site vigorously.

"Are you going to sew the lip?" I ask Dr. Swami.

"The problem is, it's full of maggots."

"Oh!"

"They are leaving today. We will just kill the maggots, give antibiotics and follow-up medication. Maybe we could stitch tomorrow, but they are leaving."

"Will it heal in a normal shape?"

"No. There is a gap. The lip will —" He makes a drooping gesture.

"Can it still eat?"

"Oh yes. It will heal."

I shake Dr. Swami's hand and press my hands together in a namaste gesture to the older man in the tent. I look at the camels lying calmly in the dirt.

It seems like such a clear choice. Stay, get a simple treatment, and make your camel look good. Why not?

But for the nomads, it is time to leave Pushkar. Staying for the sake of a single camel is not possible. The rhythms of their lives, their travels through the hills and byways, dictate that some things must be left unresolved. The group must move; there is grass and forest to be nibbled and water to be sipped. The keepers of the camels, followers of Pabuji, will move on now.

We are no different. I must go too — to Netha's village, to see Raika life up close.

31 | RAIKA VILLAGE

"Raika peoples no is cruel."
— NETHA RAIKA

Skimming down a highway in Rajasthan feels like flying in contrast to Jaipur's city traffic. Trucks decorated with riotous flower patterns pass, their horns blowing musical notes. My driver, like all the drivers I've encountered, has a shrine on the dashboard, this one consisting of a black-and-white photo of a man among tiny marigolds and powder markings. "Who is that?" I ask him, thinking it's a deceased relative. "My guru," he says.

We pass cotton fields bursting with fluffy white bolls, henna fields, dusty truck stops, and shimmering cooking fires. Netha speaks to the driver. "We going here," he says to Tony and me.

The road to Pichiyak branches off the highway, narrowing to dirt paths with white stone walls. This is Netha's village.

I expect a very rural, undeveloped place. Netha had invited us to spend the night, but having escaped a rich man's neglected Punjabi guest room at midnight a few years back because of thick dust, a flooded bathroom, and an ancient plywood bed, I didn't want to take the risk, so I opted for a day trip.

Young kids pop up from behind the walls, waving to us. In sort of a cul-de-sac, we park in the dirt under a tree. We enter Netha's family home; the driver has comfortably invited himself along. It's a huge multistory, marble-floored house. The cool, high-ceilinged living room has a shelf holding group portraits of his locally illustrious family. "My uncle is police official," says Netha modestly.

Inside sit Netha's mother and his young wife, with a cluster of small children. His mother wears a ruffled dress and the thick white elbow-to-shoulder bracelets deemed uniform by traditional Raika male herders. Everyone is barefoot. Huge sacks of lentils and rice lean against the wall. We remove our shoes and sit down. Over tea we exchange gifts; they've made me an elaborate wall hanging, three maroon circles with mirrors and a bead fringe. Netha leads us through the spacious courtyard to see the ornate guesthouse his family has just built for tourists. Our bare feet pass over floors and staircases of richly veined marble in tones of purple and cinnabar. New mattresses (hard but pristine) lie on sturdy new beds. I guess I should have said yes to his offer.

"Adams-ji, you like to visit my family out with sheep?"

Dry yellow stalks wave like wheat as we drive deep into flat grassland and park by a fence. Netha leads Tony and me through the brush and grass to a place where gray-white sheep are grazing. Near a lean-to made of sticks and leaves, two women are sitting on the ground. As we approach, they stand. "This is my family womens," says Netha. We exchange nods and smiles and take curious stock of each other. They wear colorful ruffled dresses with pink veils; I'm comparatively drab in shapeless blue pants and a yellow top. They wave me inside the hut. One opens a powder-blue cabinet and tilts a round metal pot of milk toward me. Oval shapes bob in the white. "Sheep milk with curd," says Netha. Rounds of speckled bread with blackened edges lie on a metal platter.

"They are here for long time, taking care sheep," Netha says. "They go back after six months." The place has a roof and abuts a small concrete platform with two woven cots and a well.

"Will you eat?" Netha says. "They want to cook for you."

Will we eat? Oh yes, we will. Never would I turn down a nomad meal.

"You will, Adams-ji?" He is surprised. "You no have to."

"Why not?"

"Most peoples they maybe would not."

I move into the hut as they crouch by the stone firepit. The nearest woman squats and efficiently pats out the pale-brown rotis, made from millet, and throws the rounds on the fire. As they thicken and curl in the heat, she brings out a stick of honey-brown jaggery, a form of raw sugar. The baked rotis are crumbled with the jaggery on a metal tray. Then comes ghee, the golden clarified butter. Their lithe hands, with enviably long nail beds, knead the mixture into a lumpy mass. A pot of cinnamon-brown lentils appears.

"You sit, please," says Netha, indicating the cot outside on the platform. One knee folded on the bed, my hair blown by the breeze, I accept the tray and lift a heap of the mixture to my lips. It's cake-sweet and delicious. The combination of butter, sugar, and the rich millet taste, with a hint of fire, makes me want to eat more and more.

"Now you have roti," Netha says. The crusty roti bursts with natural flavor. The women offer Netha the metal pot of sheep curd. "You want this?"

I know that raw sheep milk and curd present a risk: the natural antibacterial properties of raw milk may not compensate for contamination in handling and storage, and local germs these women's systems are primed for may bother me. But I dip a shred of roti into the pot of white bubbles and dredge up a soft oval of curd. Netha offers the lentils. A scoop of lentil, a puddle of milky curd quivering on the roti, and a chunk of the sweet concoction make a fulfilling meal.

The women come tentatively closer, watching to see if I like it. "This is so very, very good. I am honored that you make this for me." Netha sighs and says they are very pleased. The women and I make small talk with his help, watching each other as he translates.

"Your dress is beautiful," I say to one woman. It's a pieced print fabric with a gathered bodice. "Where do you get it?"

"Her daughter make very good clothes. She can make one for you, if you like."

"I would love that. But we have no time for fitting." If only I had known.

The sheep make snuffling noises in the pen. A boy shepherd on the fence says nothing as we enter the field. The animals scamper together in a defensive group. By the fence a newborn lamb lies on its side, its gray tongue visible in its narrow-toothed muzzle. "It's sick," I say.

"Yes," confirms Netha. It's too far gone to even pant for air.

"How long has it been like this?"

"Ten days."

"Why didn't they put it out of its misery, just end its life?"

"Killing is wrong," Netha says. "Raika peoples no is cruel."

Tony gets his water bottle and pours it over the open mouth. "Don't!" I say. "You're just making it suffer longer."

We watch its stiff white body. Nothing moves. Then it bleats piteously. The young shepherd picks it up and moves it to the group. The sheep back away as one. Nothing can restore it to communal life. To the flock, it's already dead. I imagine it making its passage along the great way, a darkening field, dreaming, perhaps, of being back inside its mother.

Back at the lean-to, Netha pulls a smooth leaf from a twiggy shrub. It's the lightly veined green of a praying mantis. "This is aak," he says. "We drinking camel milk from this leaf." Aak leaves are said by some to be poisonous, but they're also the only leaves the camels don't eat, and as such, they make handy nomad cups. Also, Raika people think aak has medicinal qualities when combined with camel milk. The freshly broken end weeps a latex-like sap. They take a drop of this with no ill effects, though more of it can induce vomiting. An Indian wildlife expert told me aak is used in Ayurvedic medicine to treat skin, spleen, respiratory, and gastric problems and as an antidote to snakebite.

"Adams-ji, hold it in the hand." He pinches the velvety oval leaf from underneath, shaping it into a finger-size funnel. There are no camels here, so I don't get to drink milk from the leaf.

Our time here is drawing to a close, but I don't want to leave. The day has been a muted rainbow of green and yellow leaves and the pink, blue, and mauve of the women's dresses. We smile at each other, wordlessly enjoying each other's company. One of the women beams at me with lively eyes. She's fun. We'd have so much to say to each other if we had words. But I may never pass this way again, and she may never leave this rural region. The chances of her flying are probably zero.

This outdoor world looks hard but lovely. The women know cold and heat and discomfort, but they also have cool water and smartphones and nice homes to visit on special days. They may have nice homes of their own, for all I know. They have nail polish, good tailoring, and tangy animal milk. There is birth and there is death. Not so different from my world.

We three women stand for a photo. Their bracelets are as white as their twig-cleaned teeth. My pink dupatta skims my shoulders awkwardly — nothing like theirs, centuries of grace falling capably down their backs. We make the smiling faces that say goodbye, nice to know you. And the road again leads me from a place I'd like to stay.

32 RAIKA COME IN FROM THE COLD (AND I COLLAPSE)

"You see how they are?"
— DOCTOR TO TONY

Back on the highway among the decorated trucks, we travel many hours to get to Ilse's camel festival. It's not a giant affair like the one in Pushkar, but it's solely devoted to camel herders and their causes. In the remote Rajasthani village of Sadri, we bump and bounce past Raika men and women herding camels, sheep, and cattle. We wend our way down a dirt road past breezy fields and turn in to the home of Camel Charisma, Ilse's nonprofit organization. The facility is appointed with brick and grass huts, a large white house, and an outdoor lavatory with water fountain (a scarce amenity). This week, Raika and world advocates for pastoralist people are coming here for events including dancing, a film festival, promotion of camel products, and perplexing discussions.

Atop the rambling house belonging to Ilse and her partner, Hanwant, is a rooftop café set up with cushions. I carry up a plate of soft white camel cheese and chat with photographers, filmmakers, scientists, and policy experts from India and other countries. Helping out is the impishly handsome Magan Raika, a local Raika camel advocate and herder. I've seen his thousand-watt smile on Facebook. Speaking English is hardly necessary with so much goodwill.

A huge purple and gold tent is set up for a buffet dinner. The Raika

191

men (unaccompanied by any Raika women) sit apart, majestic in their turbans and cloaks, and they are the first in line. There are metal plates, metal cups, and drinking water from a reportedly safe source.

As it grows dark, Hanwant welcomes the crowd. Dark-haired, dashing, and stocky in jeans and a casual shirt, he's a respected Rajput local from the same clan as the maharaja of Jodhpur, Gaj Singh II, who will visit the festival.

"We have special performance," Hanwant says. "The Bhopa will present the story of how Pabuji born and how brings camels to Rajasthan." The Bhopa are wandering minstrels who perform a special, almost ministerial function among the Raika: they are performers, knowledge keepers, and decision-makers. The whole performance consists of thousands of memorized verses, and Hanwant says it usually takes as long as seven nights, but we're getting a slice of the story. I've never dreamed of seeing an enactment of the Raika's cherished oral history.

Pabuji is a god revered by local herders. He was reportedly a land-lord or noble. "Pabuji went to place now in Pakistan area," Hanwant patiently explains to me in the back of the tent. "At that time Raika not know about female camels, they only know male camels. So Pabuji and some Raika and Bhopa went and they bring back female camels to Raika." That's when the Raika started breeding camels. But Pabuji returned, forsaking his own wedding to fight enemies who took his northern compatriots' cows. "He go and he died there, for the cow," Hanwant says sadly. So Pabuji is a deity now, with his own lengthy legend.

Two turbaned men and a figure in a purple and gold sari and dupatta take their places on a white cloth. The men play flat stringed instruments with curved bows, hung with jingling bells, that make a rhythmic plucking sound. Resembling lutes, they're called *ravanhattas*. The red-turbaned man in a silver necklace emits a yelp from high in his throat, reminding me of the mountain bluegrass of home. The dancer lifts her braceleted arms high, leaning back to shake them at the ceiling. She jumps sideways in a half squat, then whirls around re-peatedly as the strings and bells play on. The more I watch, the more

I notice — there's something different about the dancer. Long, hard arms; strong, straight legs. An angular torso under the sari. I can't see her face — or his face. Turns out, it's a man. I don't know the rules of this enthralling performance, but he greatly increases its charm.

After the dance, Magan drives me and other women to our hotel. He suddenly pulls over in the dark, tells them, "Wait here," and waves me out of the car. Inside a low building, in a dark and intimate space, men sing and play instruments, apparently in worship. People are seated on the ground. I crouch in the back as they pray and chant. "This my temple," says Magan. He brings me forward. The first priest speaks and places a garland of marigolds gently over my head. "He is honor you for your work helping people," Magan says. "It is good thing." He beams his radiant smile. The other women join us and are welcomed as well. Back in my room, I lay the fragrant flowers on my bed. It's the greatest acknowledgment I've ever had.

Next day we make an early start with the camel herders. With Magan at the wheel of another jeep, we bounce violently down a red-brown road. By a low green tree in a yellowing field stand a camel and a slim, handsome, bearded Raika man in a fitted white jacket with bows. He wears a red turban, and gold-milled earrings hang from his lobes. He looks familiar, standing elegantly on one muscular leg, balancing a pot on one knee. His camel has no halter. There's a red cord hobbling the forefeet, plus a belly strap and a fabric sling at the udder. His hands work the teats as the milk shoots easily out, while the camel stands re-laxed, mouthing the air. The herder smiles as he pours the frothing white milk into a bigger pot, and I recognize him. He's Bhanwarlal Raika, whose picture I've seen on the Camel Charisma website.

More herders arrive, their brown and sand-colored camels also hobbled for milking. A dark, gangly baby camel, thin as a knife blade, mewls and barks as it peers around its mom. Babies suckle from one teat as the herder milks the other; meanwhile, the camel mothers munch greenery in a bucolic tableau.

Bhanwarlal finishes milking and joins us cross-legged on the ground with Magan (they are probably distant relatives, although Magan calls him by the common title *Uncle*). Smiling, Bhanwarlal heats water on the fire to make a narcotic tea. "*Afyom*," Magan says — the herders have it every morning. He holds a cup of the mocha liquid out to me. I have to speak at the festival today, so I drink very little and feel no effects.

As more Raika men join us, Magan puts his face right next to a camel's and kisses it. His blazing white smile beguiles me to try. I walk slowly over, quaveringly placing my lips near the camel's. But I fear getting bitten. I worry that my hesitation may confuse the camel, and so I pull back.

"Whaaaat, why you no kiss camel?" Magan asks, but I just wave him off and admit that I'm a puzzle.

Back at Camel Charisma, I get out of the jeep. A tall, commanding, thick-browed man in a mustard shirt and a yellow-gold turban says, "Welcome. I am T. K. Gahlot." He places a hardback book on camel research into my hands, smiling warmly. Dr. Gahlot! He's a renowned camel surgeon. Since I now have many Indian herder connections, I've referred cases of sick camels to him. But we've never communicated, and I didn't think he knew I existed. He's driven from Bikaner, home to the Indian camel research center, where he treats problems in all manner of beasts. I feel honored to be met by him. And now the camel festival begins.

A vast pale-blue tent, draped with white and pink ruched curtains, holds rows of chairs, with white sofas for honored guests placed on and below the stage. A statue of Pabuji, adorned with flowers, makes a tabletop shrine. Herders arrive en masse, the men in white clothes, ornate gold jewelry, and top-shaped red turbans that outnumber the pink and gold ones. I see dark eyes and mustaches, walking sticks and weathered faces, a full white beard blooming here and there. Musicians start playing the lively, jangling tunes of last night. Ilse, practical in pants and a sleeveless quilted vest, invites me to sit in the front row. A government minister in a gold turban and khaki uniform arrives.

"Welcome to the Marwar Camel Festival," Ilse says onstage, the microphone echoing through the tent. "We have camel herders here from Jaisalmer, Udaipur, and cities all over Rajasthan to discuss their problems and the state of the camels. And people from other countries, to join in." Men circle the Pabuji shrine as she speaks, lighting the candles and arranging the marigolds. "We have to show there is *potential* of the camel — and we have to make *use* of it if we want to save it," she continues in German-accented English.

Behind me the Raika men listen quietly, seeming morose or worried. Dr. Gahlot joins the officials on the white sofas onstage. Others sit cross-legged on the stage floor. Because the camels can't legally be sold across state lines, we discuss camel products that can: wool, leather, milk, and meat — even camel poop. Ilse's group makes thick gray paper by blending it with cotton, powder, and guar gum, and it has zero smell. Camel-hair rugs and cheese are made here too. I have camel-poop stationery in my desk back home, and I've bought a rug to take back. I know that these products would be popular with other customers, but the herders aren't technologically savvy, and Sadri is so remote that shipping isn't easy. A raging monsoon flood can trap Ilse at home, knock out her electricity, and shut down her online store.

So far camel milk is still the product of greatest interest. As the talk turns to milk, an officious man from Bikaner says onstage that his research organization uses camel milk for autism, diabetes, and tuberculosis.

I stand and tell the audience that I know of a small-business model for people who, like these herders, "stay at home with animals, don't go to much school, and live far away from cities." (I don't mention the Amish by name, because that's just too complicated.) "They are making good money," I say, rubbing my fingers together in what I hope is a universal signifier. "Parents of children with autism are a big driver of the market in the world." A young woman translates my words into Hindi: *unt* (camel) and *dudh* (or *doodh*, milk). "If you provide very clean milk, hygienically handled, with good testing, you can develop a loyal customer base." I'm glad to see the men are listening, because who knows what cultural norms I may be violating with my recommendations. After all, they have refused to sell camel milk, wool, or female camels before now. "These customers are sick people, and they don't want buffalo or goat milk mixed in, as it can hurt them," I caution, and a Raika in a twisted white turban nods at that. Knowing that cellphones are central to personal and business interactions in India, I add, "If someone can help you reach these customers on social media or by phone, you can develop a relationship. Thank you for the value you offer the world," I say, then bow slightly and sit down.

From behind me a beedi appears, passed by some Raika men. I take it, breathe in the smoke, and get a pleasantly swimming head. Tony is shocked. "I have to get a picture, the kids won't believe it!" he says.

That night, I lie on the rose-print duvet on our pushed-together twin beds. I'm hot, then cold, and I barely sleep. But I get up in the morning and put on my new red *salwar* trimmed with lace. I'm giving my own presentation at noon.

Outside the blue tent, a camel stands to welcome us, draped in a cloak of many bright colors. There seems to be some sort of electrical crisis in the tent. And I'm not doing well. "Hey, do you feel okay?" I ask everyone. They've had the same food and drinks as I did. And it's been several days since I had the sheep milk.

"Yes, lovely, thank you," they reply, with puzzled looks. I go to lie down in Ilse and Hanwant's round brick hut (they've lent their house to guests), staring at the thatched roof point where the grass tips form a peak. Soon it's time to get up; the show must go on. They've moved my talk to a golden tent glowing with printed motifs.

Families from cities start to arrive. One autistic boy of nine has a clubfoot and cannot speak but has keened the same tune for three long years. "It drives me mad in the car sometimes," confides his adoring dad. He's feisty, this shaven-headed, mischievous boy, and a master at getting his way. I tell his lovely, sad-eyed parents about possible therapies and doctors as he hums and tugs them endlessly, lunging in all directions. This child's needs are placing the whole family at risk, but there's only one faraway pediatric neurologist, with a six- to twelve-month wait list. In all cultures, in families of kids with autism, suicide, divorce, abandonment, and even child murder happen. Support for the family is important, as well as therapy for the child.

Unlike American autism meetings, this event has attracted many men and fathers. There are doctors from Bikaner and herders from the field. Soon the seats fill up, and a line starts to form. The organizers put a loudspeaker outside as the sunlight filters through the gold.

Raika men file in, looking resplendent today, like buccaneers, with their mustaches and gold shield necklaces. Some refuse the chairs and settle on the floor in front. The rest sit or stand in back. They talk to a few other Indian men but mainly keep to themselves.

I ask the man next to me, "Can you translate?" He's a doctor and says yes.

In my slide presentation, I use short sentences to keep the concepts simple. I show pictures of Marlin and his family, and camels from other countries. The Raika look closely at these faraway but familiar images. Families sit next to vets, herders beside policy makers. This is the inter-laced community we need to help preserve camels and camel culture. When my talk is over, parents and science folks come up to chat. Ilse's happy. I stand and speak with journalists and pose for family pictures.

Then suddenly I feel like fainting. I slip away to the hut again. There's a twist in my organs and I come undone. I go to the lavatory and throw up, then lie back down. When Magan comes to check on me, his face drops in concern, and he goes to fetch Tony and Hanwant. I ask for a local doctor, but Ilse doesn't know one in town. "What a hardy constitution she's developed," I marvel, since she's written about a similar sickness she had when she arrived.

Over the next few hours, I feel much worse. Magan returns with someone he identifies as a doctor. The man presses my arm and at first predicts my illness will pass. He, Tony, and Magan peer down at me, now so weak I feel I'm sinking into the mattress. "Take her to the hospi-tal? Clinic?" he says — now he's alarmed. Magan commandeers some-one's jeep, and after a nightmare trip in the back seat, Tony hauls me up the steps of what looks like a small village store. Scattered young peo-ple look casually at my wrinkled clothes and thin down jacket. Inside the tiny clinic, they gesture to two ancient, leathery exam tables, their tops cracked like tortoiseshells, without curtains or protective paper. I lie down, shivering and burning in waves. Then two men, a boy, and a woman enter. A man takes the chair two feet away.

The doctor arrives. He asks for a medical history, and Tony starts to give it, but since this is serious, I add details that might matter. "I'm sensitive to medications and don't need a lot, I'm allergic to contrast dye and don't process B vitamins well," I croak out.

He looks at his assistant and holds his hands out in frustrated amusement. "You see?" he says. "You see how they are?" Tony laughs with him as I lie huddled on my side. "They know so much, their standards are so high." He smiles and his eyes soften as he considers me. "We must put you in the hospital, you are very dehydrated. We have to run tests." He lists some of them: dengue, malaria, cholera. Others he only hints at, trying not to scare me.

"I think it's just food poisoning." Usually I take precautions, and they have always worked. Still, I've been exposed to truck-stop food en route to Ilse's, dishes washed in uncertain water, and other potential sources of illness. And there's been a lethal virus going around. Although I'm normally pretty tough, I'm horrifically sick now.

He makes a decision. "We can do this where you don't go to the hospital — I think. Call me if you feel much worse, but it should be fine." He gives Tony a raft of medicines with exact dosing schedules and prescribes constant cold sponge baths to bring my fever down. Now it's time for a shot and blood work.

"Original packaging for needles?" I say faintly, as politely as I can. I know a hepatitis C outbreak once got started with reused needles in an Indian village. He looks at me like I'm crazy. "We do that everywhere now." He comes close and motions me to pull down the side of my pants. The waiting man and boy watch expressionlessly, like they're at a ball game.

"Tony, hold up my jacket," I say, to block them. Why do *I* have to think of this? I get a shot and collapse again.

I stumble out, grateful for the aid of this intuitive and competent man. The visit, medicines, and tests cost the equivalent of seven US dollars. If we could only do so well back home.

After a night of extraordinary misery and shiver-inducing sponge baths, in the morning I'm exhausted but alive. Few people at the festival know what happened to me; I asked Magan to keep it quiet so as not to distract from the program. "Today is the maharaja's visit," I say, dismayed. He's a major cultural supporter. I'll miss the pomp and pageantry of his arrival, because I'm still too damn sick to even get to the door. Then there's a knock. Tony answers. A family has come to see me.

I get myself shakily together and meet them in the yard. Sitting in a circle with two brothers and their wives, we talk about their autistic nephew in America. They love him so much that they tracked me down at my hotel. I'm glad they aren't bothered by my wan and crumpled face. I give them names and numbers, a suggestion for a plan. They leave, so sweet and gracious, with new hope for his future.

Sitting alone in the grass, I stare at the pool. I swam there with pleasure two days in a row. On those afternoons, the birds called, the breeze blew, flowers nodded over the clear water. It was nirvana. Now this may have been, and could still be, the worst illness of my life.

I slump in the chair to think it over. Right now I want to go home. But I've felt the sun, walked the fields, and heard the jangling camels. I've done something bigger than myself, tried to help an ancient culture. Many explorers have died while pursuing their goals. If I'd died here, at least I would have reached one of mine. If that's not worth living for, then dying doesn't matter.

After I recover and head to my other events, Dr. Ilse sends word that the festival was a success. The government has granted formal permission to sell camel milk and may offer more support. The valiant Raika herders may have gained a second chance.

33 LIFE IN "THE SAND"

"But their knowledge is also science — it is more than science."
— Dr. Abdul Raziq Kakar

"Allaaah..." The drone of a prayer call floats over the dust of the camel souk. It's evening, and the great orange sun that warmed us a moment ago is sinking. In a corner of Al Ain, a city in Abu Dhabi on the border with Oman, I'm surrounded by hundreds of camels. Wide-chested black Saudi males, lean grayish racers, and brown, ecru, almond, and patchwork camels with blue eyes stand in roomy stalls.

The hazy light over the boxy beige buildings doesn't dim the lively, dark eyes of Dr. Abdul Raziq Kakar. We've never spoken until today, but we've communicated for years, trading camel lore and knowledge. A veterinary science professor from Pakistan, he is technical operations manager at the local Al Ain Farms, which offers camel milk along with other food and dairy products. Raziq is a student of plants, earth, animals, and ecosystems. Stricken a few years ago with a form of arthritis so crippling he couldn't walk, he took camel milk and recovered completely. With cropped black hair, dressed in fashionable jeans and a striped polo shirt, he gives an impression of tireless vigor. In addition, he's a huge camel-milk advocate (he's one of many men who say it enhances virility).

On a stopover in Dubai on my way home from India, I've driven nearly a hundred miles to meet him. In the camel souk, dressed in a blue-yellow tunic, leggings, and mirrored blue dupatta, I feel sand creeping into my sandals. Similarly sandaled workers from Somalia, Sudan, Afghanistan, and Pakistan walk by, in long white tunics called *kandura*, or tunic-and-pants sets in solid gray or burgundy called *salwar kameez*. All wear head wraps and caps.

"When I first came here to Al Ain, I came to the souk every Saturday. The people working here were friend to me, and I learned from them, especially the hot branding," Raziq says, touching his forearm. Branding is an ethnic medicinal treatment. "These people, they have traditional knowledge about camel — how to care, to treat, make it healthy, strong." He points toward the pens as a bird lands with a flutter. "We witness in the last ten, twenty years that science says, no, this is wrong, this is true, this is wrong. But *their* knowledge is processed through ages — one thousand, two thousand years. I am scientist and I believe in science. But their knowledge is also science — it is *more* than science."

This is not an outlandish statement in the Rub' al Khali (the Empty Quarter), the largest continuous sand desert in the world, stretching over Saudi Arabia, Yemen, Oman, and the United Arab Emirates. Bedouins call it simply "the sand." Al Ain is a fertile oasis at the edge of the desert, a place where traders have stopped to water their camels for millennia. Home to United Nations World Heritage and other archaeological sites from the Bronze and Neolithic ages, it is now a city with over half a million residents. Copper, pearls, and dates were once traded here. Today Al Ain retains its rich desert heritage, intentionally limiting skyscrapers and opening old forts and palaces to the public.

We stroll toward the pens, Tony along with us. A pale camel, covered in a gray print blanket with a black tuft of hair peeking from the top, appears to smile as a taller camel nuzzles its face. (Scientists aren't convinced they really smile, but herders often think so. And camel vocalizations are perceived as very emotive by their keepers.) Their heads turn away, looking like they've made a secret agreement to meet. "That is racing camel," says Raziq. All kinds of camels are for sale here: families come to buy camels for milking, others buy them for meat or racing. An abattoir lies conveniently across the yard. "But this souk is *speshall*," says Raziq. This is one of his favorite words, and it's delightful to hear him say it, with his elegantly elongated *sh*'s.

I can close my eyes and imagine it's one thousand years ago, and around me people are hawking camels for sale. "These people use traditional knowledge to care for and sell it. They can explain the beauty of the camels to you. A layperson cannot see it," he says. But I can see it — and hear it. The noise of camels swishing placidly through their fodder, with their peculiar stillness even in motion, the cooling air, the occasional grunts and groans across the roomy pens, make this a place of peace. The camels are brokered and boarded by locals and out-of-towners from Oman and Dubai. But some people, Raziq tells me, choose to live on site as caretakers. "Many people stay here, because they like it — they like the smell, the..."

Here comes the racing camel again, led by a man in a white tunic and flat cap. "How much is that camel?" asks Raziq, but the man is not in the mood to chat. Over his shoulder I see a group of male workers kneeling in the lot for evening prayers.

Raziq leads us to a dirt and concrete rise, where the camels are loaded on and off trucks, sometimes in slings. "Wherever I went," he says, recalling his travels before his arrival not long ago, "I chose one tree as my friend." He gestures to the only tree in sight. "This tree is very speshall, she is my friend." It's a local acacia with wind-shaped branches. Clinging to the bone-dry dirt, it's nearly hollow and tied with a cotton rag. How it remains upright is a miracle. "This place is from thousands of years ago. You can see the resistance of this tree, in this hard place, with no water, nothing. She is happy, she is giving shade."

"Did you give her a name?" I ask.

"Souk tree," he says, bending over the trunk. "She is alive — this is her power of resistance."

Two young workers ask for a photo with us. I take pictures of them with Raziq and Tony, but the wiry young guy with dimples wants one with me and the other worker. I stand in the middle, smiling, holding my hands out in a fun pose, when I feel his hand slip around my waist, then knead and grope my hip like a loaf of bread dough. *Little creep!* I think.

It's not the first time. On my first trip to India, a sales clerk in a dressing room groped me as he adjusted the fit of my long dress. Tony had been waiting outside, but that didn't matter. The clerk was fired after we informed the manager. But now I'm faced with a choice. Do I say something and blow this whole situation up? In an Islamic country where even public hand-holding can earn an onlooker's scolding? I don't want to get the man imprisoned for years — he's still a kid, if an impudent, obnoxious one. And I wonder if he's poor and far away from home, living in a camel souk. Anger, fear, and empathy clash in my mind. I don't want to embarrass my host, and I have no time to stay for court proceedings. No one else notices what he did. The little brat. *Let him have my hip*, I think, sighing with tired resentment, and walk on.

We wander among the camels, noting their characteristics. It's too dark for me to make out more than shapes now, but Raziq is not fazed. "That is an Omani camel. His daughter will be a good milker." The camel moans, making blub-blub-blub sounds.

"How can you tell?"

"It's his shape, his head, his configuration. I can close my eyes and take the skin of the camel in my fingers and tell which part of the world it is from, *inshallah*." He strokes the camel intimately, like a pet. "I have one thousand years' experience, because I took the experience of the people who have one thousand years' experience!"

Raziq has traveled to forty-six countries and lived with nomads in mountains and desert sand for his research. "They are the treasures of knowledge, believe me." He found the people easy to communicate with. "Some people talk and make another face than what they are thinking," he says, but this experience helps him sense a person's inner being. By contrast, "There is no double standard in the animals," he says. He's not a fan of progress that excludes nomadic lives. "The US and Pakistan, we built roads and bridges, but we lost our vista."

We peek briefly into the abattoir. Meat is an important part of the camel economy in Africa and the Middle East. It's very lean and nutritious, viewed as a curative in itself. An ideal Ramadan feast features a whole roasted camel, on a giant platter with rice and vegetables — not something you'd do with a twenty-five-thousand-dollar American camel but maybe affordable here. I chat with the friendly young veterinarian who runs the place. A skinned camel hangs behind me, its flesh red-purple.

According to Raziq, the Bedouins are now wealthy enough to sell the old and injured camels they once ate. They dispose of theirs here and buy fresh yearlings or two-year-olds for meat. "Look around," he says. "Ninety-nine percent are young people, poor people, they need meat." These folks boil the tough old camels for a curry sauce. "Indian and other peoples, they eat. Pashtun and Sudani people, they are meat lovers." The young camels make a good pilau (rice dish), Raziq adds.

While this makes the camels sound like any meat livestock, they evolved as a free-ranging animal, with unique needs. Raziq describes their special yet delicate musculature as we stand in the gloom, singling out camels to illustrate his points. They can get injured by modern handlers who don't have traditional training. "If they are not exercised, and you just start fresh and pull on them," it may harm a muscle, he explains. Before, "they were roaming, eating good plants to remedy their injuries." But today's camels don't always get to do this, making them less hardy than their "ship of the desert" reputation suggests.

In the darkened wire cages, amid grunts and blubbers, our hands trace the sides, noses, and curved backs of warm-haired camels. This place of cyclic life and death is still beautiful, an oasis of survival. I tear myself away from their wide-eyed faces, and we climb into the SUV to leave.

The sounds of past centuries grow fainter as I look back at the old souk tree. She's endured the indignities of a thousand years, the piss and shit of camels and men; she's been torn by wind, bumped by trucks, deprived of even a drink. But she lives on with no visible help, surviving in her silence.

Raziq brings us to his home. We remove our shoes and sit on layers of beautiful carpets. His children bring out platters arrayed with cut cucumbers and tomatoes, a bowl of meat on the bone, a yogurt dish, and round chapati-style bread, then return with shyly confident smiles to the kitchen where his wife cooks. She does not join us. I know

Raziq is very fond of her, as we have texted about her health before she joined him from Pakistan. He, Tony, and I eat and share stories. "Here is speshall shawl made from soft white wool, by a camel friend. Here is a drawing by my daughter," he says. After dinner I (but not Tony) am invited into the warm and steamy kitchen, where I compliment his rosy-faced wife on the feast. "My wife is very good cook," says Raziq. The dinner plates she and the children have used sit on a small table. We smile at each other in appreciation.

We spend that night at another Rotana hotel: there's an architecturally tall gold tea set in the lobby, set in the hush of elegant Muslim hospitality. No livestock smell, no dust; it's a different kind of oasis, independent of time and space. Outside lies Oman, an orange-red landscape that lures me to the window next morning before Raziq picks us up.

We wind through the sunny city's roundabouts. It's as modern and carefully laid out as a planned California community, with smooth streets, wide roads, and fringed vegetation waving subtly in the wind. Our destination is the opposite of yesterday's ancient souk: the huge food processing operation of Al Ain Farms. Outside the gates, we enter a factory free of any speck of desert dust. In a large warehouse, sacks of white powder are stacked on pallets: camel milk.

It's strangely comforting to fly across the world and see milk you've cooked with at home. I've used this powdered milk in tea and smoothies, and made mashed potatoes for my kids with it (two of the girls can't tolerate other dairy). The small blue packets I'd sampled were filled with these same featherweight flakes. Al Ain is trying to figure out how to market the milk, which is just one of their many product lines. Started by Sheikh Zayed in the 1980s with a herd of two hundred cows, it has grown into a major purveyor of cow milk, juices, poultry, and now camel milk. I see the processing equipment in the factory and meet the welcoming management and staff, who hail from South Asia, Europe, and other parts of the world.

We climb into another SUV and head out to see the camels. An oxidized swath of soft red sand, wavy with camel tracks, is dotted with about 1,700 fit, grayish-brown camels, some with black tufts or silky neck fringes. They stand or laze about pad-deep in the sand, or knees down in a relaxed cush position. Moos, groans, and burbles float from airy side lots that hold more camels Tony, Raziq, and I are here with regal young farm manager, Mubarak, who's immaculate in a starched, head-to-toe white collarless kandura, with a matching white ghutra draping his head and shoulders. We get out and take it all in.

Across the powdery sand we walk, under a bright-blue sky. In a lightly fenced and shaded enclosure I see four or five baby camels. A young farmworker lets me in. Looking around, I spot more, kneeling or standing in the corners, fourteen elegant young camels, in charcoal, vanilla, and tobacco, solid-colored and ombre, their humps tipped with fluffy black tufts. I hold my finger out for them to sniff. Like little ballet dancers, they step closer on their spindly legs, lifting long, bony noses to the air. Their curly coats are as soft as sheep pelts.

"Mehhhh, mowwww, muhhh," they bleat. Their tails swish sideways like wipers on a car as they explore the strange mother in their midst. The worker gives me a bottle of camel milk. A cashew-colored baby reaches for the nipple, left leg en pointe, and I tip the bottle downward as it suckles, smacking its lips.

Two stand closer. One samples my leg like an uncertain delicacy, then extends its head around to peer at my back. Another presses for a taste with a "mehhhh." He runs his face down me, chest to leg, then pushes his nose into my blouse. A dark, marble-eyed baby comes for a sip of milk, and walks away moaning, white drops hanging from whiskers and lashes. Joy washes over me. Their inquisitive faces, their doll lashes and hooked necks, their sudden gamboling, make them seem like playthings come to life.

These babies are kept here after birth with their moms to give them a healthy start in life. Camels here can give up to fifteen liters of milk daily after birth, so there's more than enough to keep the babies happy and fill bottles for the dairy. Moms give milk for up to thirteen months. Then it's time to make babies once again.

I tear myself away from the nuzzling and mooing, the grunting and kissing. Camel therapy for humans would be a wondrous thing, worth hundreds for a session. By the fence, Raziq absently strokes a baby's throat as he smiles and chats with the men, his hands gently encircling its neck.

Raziq and Mubarak show us around the rest of the lot. Camels are doing their camelid duties (standing, chatting, ambling). A tall, friendly camel joins our little group. Raziq and Mubarak point to its neck, which holds an embedded chip and a numbered collar that identifies it to the Abu Dhabi government and the Al Ain system. This good-natured beast is dotted with several circle-shaped scars. "It's *wasum*," says Raziq. This form of branding is used for tribal identification, but also as a medical treatment for humans and animals: a hot metal rod is applied to the part of the body thought to be the site of the problem.

"Is that to provoke an immune response?" I ask Raziq.

"Yes, bring blood rushing," he says.

"But we have more," says Mubarak, his full lips framed by his neat beard. "I *know*. We have camel racing, we have one hundred camels," he says with the casual assurance of his family heritage. "Before I am children, we have pain" — he presses his upper stomach — "and we put one side there," indicating his left side, "and three there," he says, tapping his upper back three times.

"It's like acupuncture," says Raziq. "With iron, put in fire until it's red."

"For babies born small, that go into the glass, how do you say it?" Mubarak asks.

"The incubator," I say.

"Yes, when they have blue body and eyes have color..."

"Yellow?"

"Ya," he says.

"That's jaundice."

"Yes, for jaundice, we touch it there and there" — he touches his own inner wrist and above the crook of his elbow — "and no more problem, is fine."

"This camel has an ugly toe problem," I say. Its bones are showing through the eaten-away footpad.

"If we have pain in the forehand, like here" — he points to the ragged front foot — "we touch to different part of here and here" — he traces a line below the camel's ear — "and in three days, no more problem."

This particular camel's obviously feeling no pain, because it's fresh in love with Tony. Mooning, smiling, looming over my man, it's besotted, like a boyfriend offering a wilted rose. Tony pats it, and it follows us toward the SUV, our twelve legs shushing through glowing copper sand in a real-life caravan.

"How do you keep this sand so nice?" I ask Raziq.

"We clean it every day. With a sand cleaner" — like the ones used for beaches, he explains. "Spray every day, to keep the flies down. The sand is changed every six months, then whole new sand," Raziq explains.

We guiltily leave the lovestruck camel and drive toward the milking area. A row of camels stands behind a simple pole fence, eating from a concrete trough. They're fed a blend of fiber, alfalfa, corn, soy, grasses, and other nutrients, slightly different from Al Ain cow feed. "Cow is grass eater, camel is bush eater," says Raziq, as a male voice on the car radio intones a hypnotic song.

"But different," says Mubarak. "Milking camels big. For racing, bodies small *here*" — he makes the shape of a torso — "but more power." Al Ain milks around 450 camels daily, depending on the season, collecting an average of eight liters per camel per day.

In the wide red sand lot, I see camels lining up at a white gate for the second milking of the day. No one is herding them. "They know what to do," I marvel. The men nod; they see it every day. As the gate opens, a stream of camels flows through. Like minnows in a creek, they glide unhurried to their destination. Full-uddered mothers with tall, sculpted bodies move together. Inside the open shed, they mill quietly around. The babies aren't needed to stimulate milking, but they are kept nearby so they can see their mothers afterward. Like those in Dubai, these camels give milk on their own.

"This is amazing, how they come so easily — and they look so happy," I whisper. Their lower lips are dropped, their rangy bodies ambling calmly; they are a tribute to the animal-human bond.

But what about the farm's twenty-four fathers-in-waiting? We drive past Bull Shed Number 1. These big boys are moved into "houses" with a group of thirty-five to forty-five female camels to breed. If pregnancies occur within four to five months, "we keep it," Mubarak says. "If not get pregnant, we put it outside and put another."

"Do they get bored, and maybe do better in a new house?" I ask. But my meaning seems lost in translation, which may be a good thing.

We pass the lab, which routinely tests the animals for disease and overall health status, and the exercise track for slightly chubby camels. There seem to be few amenities they don't have.

After a nice lunch with staff, we say our goodbyes. Raziq stops at the gate and urges us out of the car. He plucks a piece of plant growing harmlessly by the fence. "It's haram."

Forbidden? Did I hear that right?

"Harm. That is the name." Not forbidden (haram). He holds it up, ever the professor. "It's very speshall. Camels love to eat it, especially useful for moisture and salt. Or when constipation or low food intake." It's an alkaline, salt-loving species called *Zygophyllum qatarense*, he says.

He places the green branch in my hands. I twist it like a sponge, and liquid comes dripping out. It seems magical, like I've won something, and we all laugh at my surprise.

He has one last stop for us. The narrow roads to an Al Ain oasis lead through low stone walls. In a dusty lot, we park, walk a short distance, enter the brush, and step down, down into greenery. With each step, the temperature drops. Coolness settles over my sun-warmed skin. A wicked spray of thorns bobs above our heads. Fallen logs make natural bridges. Unseen water trickles and babbles among the leaves and bushes.

This is the place that camel riders dreamed of over centuries of crossing the Empty Quarter. The thought of this water, the sighing breeze, the chance to splash in a brook and wash the journey off their skin, must have kept them going. It's clear why people once fought for this site — without water, there could be no camels, and without camels, there could be no life.

For Raziq, such places are the homes of friends. He says camels eat the horrifically sharp thorns that menace our heads, nibbling with their clever articulated lips. He points out the low stone channels that funnel the water, a very old system that was used to irrigate the city's date palms. Leaves and sticks crunch under our feet as we wander in the underbrush.

Leaving the moisture-laden oasis, we walk to an old mud-walled house with a carved wooden door. Inside we see curved niches where milk and food were stored. There are no rooms or partitions, just one hardened dirt floor.

This harshly beautiful land shows the camel in perfect clarity. The camel was essential, the people's protector, the carrier and giver of goods and nutrition. And its double eyelids, the fringe of thick lashes, the long jointed legs, the crazy assemblage of hump, hair, and foot, are masterpieces of adaptation. With its long-boned nose and delicate sense of smell, it can even detect microbes that indicate the presence of water.

Here it's also clear why the camel has no natural predators. It outdoes every other creature in its ability to travel, find food, and cool itself in the desert.

The city of Al Ain still retains its past, with classic Bedouin elements: camels, humans, water, and desert. The Empty Quarter isn't empty if you know where to look. I'm richer for the lessons I've learned from Raziq and his speshall friends — the trees, rocks, and beings I've found out here in "the sand."

34 CAMEL MILK SEEKERS HAVE QUESTIONS

"It's all good."
— JONAH

Camel milk is exploding in popularity worldwide, and thousands of kids are drinking it. Science is showing that camels and their milk hold promise for human health far beyond what I'd imagined. My inbox is full, and I lecture at science conferences. People send messages from Pakistan, Morocco, Saudi Arabia, Australia, Hong Kong, Cyprus, Canada, the UAE, Kuwait, India, Greenland, Britain, France, Holland, Germany, and beyond — and from every state in the Union, big cities, small towns, and everywhere in between.

The questions from parents are always the same: "I saw your article/video online, and I want to give my son/daughter camel milk. Where can I find it? How much do I give? Bless you and thank you." After a round or two of chat, some ask, "How is your son?"

How is my son? I think about him every day, and sometimes at night when I wake.

He is fine. Okay. Not "cured," but doing astonishingly well with his life.

He can drive a car and a boat. At twenty, he's about to get his driver's license, as neither of us was in a rush. His last driving teacher turned him off — "too militaristic, a bad-cop type," he said. He skateboards, bikes, and takes trains and buses. He shares rides with friends, or his sisters and I pick him up. He can run a forklift, operate a drill, and help on a loading dock. He works part-time and takes community college classes. "You know school wasn't the easiest setting for me, so I wanted to take a break for a while." He lives in an apartment with someone to check on him and me nagging intermittently ("Clean your room, clip your nails, wash that jacket").

He's beyond bright, a big-picture thinker. He knows history, is perceptive about politics, cracks jokes on topics like memes or social-media fights. A keen observer of his peers and overall social situations, he remembers details and weaves topics into conversations. He sometimes forgets to do things (conveniently if he doesn't want to do them), but otherwise he's pretty practical. "Articulate, insightful, intellectual," Tony says. (Tony has insights into young masculinity that I don't. When I fret that Jonah hasn't called us in five days, Tony responds: "Twenty-year-old men don't always call their mothers.")

People who meet him can't tell he has autism. "You could say you have mild Asperger's in case anyone ever notices anything," I tell him. (Although that diagnosis was officially removed from the medical lineup and folded into what's now called the autism disorder spectrum, it still fits people who might not be seen as fully autistic.)

"Naw. Those are a different kind of people. I prefer to say a little bit of autism, because it's a separate thing. The people with Asperger's are kind of nonemotional and sort of controlling. That's cool, because that's just how they are. But I'm more laid back and sociable. Like, I let things go."

"Okay. Not that anyone ever asks you."

"Sometimes I just tell them offhand, like in case anything comes up," he says.

"You do?" I ask.

"Yes, it's just easier," he says, shrugging. "They're always surprised and say, I never would have known. Then they tell me about someone they know who has it but say they're a lot worse."

"Wow," I say, kind of scared for him.

"It's all good," he says, as he often does. "People are pretty chill.

Wait till you meet my new friend, you'd smell spectrum all over him, as soon as he's in your sights," he adds, with his trademark dimpled grin.

He plays second banana in a shifting guys' band. He's growing up, going out at night, having beach bonfires, and eating junk food with friends. And he's so nice.

At the end of every call, he says, "Love you," casually dropping it in. What was once the most impossible thing in the world — speaking, expressing emotion — is as common as air. His biology is something his doctor still monitors. But he eats cheese now without outward symptoms, even though I suspect it still affects him. Then again, maybe all those years of drinking camel milk alleviated the problem. He still drinks camel milk when I mix him a smoothie.

"How is the rain hitting you guys?" he asks, calling during a storm. "I heard it was coming down fast, and I don't want you to get flooded again." Impossible. Impossible that he should be calling me on the phone, thinking of other people. With every year I see more improvement. People with autism generally reach maturity later than neurotypical individuals, and development of executive function (organizational ability) takes about one-third longer. He's still working on this. But if there's something Jonah wants, he's on top of it. And he's never late to work or events — an adorable personality trait.

He knows I'm a writer. He's been writing himself. And he's well aware of my work. But he has an inner view of me as a child-oriented teacher. "What do you think of all the therapies you had?" I ask him.

"Oh, are you kidding? I'd be sitting in a room smearing stuff on the walls without them," he says, laughing. "Seriously, I get scared if I think what would have happened to me without them, and if I didn't have you. I appreciate everything you've done."

Never give up. That's a mantra in the autism community and many other places. I totally agree — and yet I don't. Giving up is often necessary. When something won't hold, no forcing will achieve it. But in the path you end up taking, there are things beyond belief. Jonah is the miracle I've always hoped for, and I'm grateful for his giving, loving grace.

35 UNTO HER A CAMEL IS BORN

"Groooo."
— APRIL, NEW MOTHER

The pregnant camel looks over her shoulder at a slender white leg waving from her extruded gray vagina, like a turtle's head poking from its shell. She's lying in Marlin's barn in Michigan, her curly brown coat picking up straw and bits of dirt. Wearing only a halter, she has her legs tucked under her, the back one slightly trembling. Her dark-brown tail tenses as a second leg emerges. The mother's eyes are open, her lips pressed together. She doesn't look perturbed, just alert. April, the daughter of Tanzania, is one of the second generation of camels to be born on Marlin's farm. Now she's giving Marlin a grandbaby camel. He's broadcasting the birth to his online friends.

"Groooo," she says, her eyes blinking twice.

Two other female camels stand five feet away in the neighboring stall, seemingly smiling, their heads craned toward her in what looks like sympathy. "Spectators!" Marlin says. "These girls are like, we just got done with it — it's possible." They look at Marlin, as if startled to be caught, and touch noses, whispering out of his earshot.

"Come on, April, push it out!" Marlin says.

The calf's grayish head slips out, its eyes peering into the straw. It sniffs, its neck wrapped tightly in the long whorl of vaginal muscle.

214

April tilts over like a top as the baby twists its head between her quivering loins.

"We're happy to see the baby is alive, and can't wait to see what sex it is," Marlin says for the video. Now April's upright again, laboring on her belly. The thin gray baby slides out with a little tug from Marlin and lies panting quickly, flat as a paper cutout. Its long, wet neck flops snakelike in the straw.

"It's a little female, which we're very excited about," Marlin says jubilantly.

Soon the mother rises, stolid against the red barn wall. She leans her giant head tenderly over the prone form. The quivering calf shuffles her own matchstick legs in the straw, exhausted from birth but eager to rise. She struggles through the dry yellow strands. "Look, the baby went sternal all on its own," Marlin says, as the newborn rolls herself upright. Milk-gray, the color of fresh snow over dirt, she flips and kicks like a deer. Her head lifts up, toward her mother, and falls backward under its own weight.

Thirty minutes after the birth, Marlin has trimmed the umbilical cord and rubbed the baby down, leaving her woolly white. Her huge eyes seem to cross over her narrow nose. April lies back down, passing the glistening blue tube of afterbirth without help. Then she rises, her muscles trembling from releasing a new life into the universe. April lets her colostrum (the first milk) flow, and after the baby gets all she wants, Marlin gathers a bit for human friends. All is well in the cozy barn.

But outside, Marlin's reluctantly making some adjustments. He finds himself doing what all pastoralists and nomads must — trying to make a natural living within unnatural boundaries. He's scraping the frozen landscape outside into a safari park to provide another use for the camels in case he tires of dealing with secular milk authorities. If pushed, he'll pack up and move to the place in America he dreads most — liberal California, where raw milk sales are less restricted and the climate is kind.

The baby is ready to nurse. Soft and white, she explores her mouth with her tongue. Her mother's udder is swollen, with stiff gray teats. April comes over, lowers her head, and nuzzles her baby's face. The sound of swishing straw and the groans and calls of camels will continue as day falls into night. The great circle of camels has grown by one. In the farm, in the world, they keep getting born.

Inshallah, they will, some cameleers would say. *God willing, may it always be so.*

AFTERWORD

The World Wakes Up to Camels

It's been years since I first met the camel in California. Now camels are the second-fastest-growing species of livestock in the world. People text me pictures of celebrities buying thirty-dollar bottles of camel milk. The Facebook camel milk group has thousands of members, and anyone can buy flash-pasteurized milk and spray-dried or freeze-dried powdered milk, which benefits many users.

Laws governing the sale of raw milk are changing. Distribution is legal in forty-three US states, serving 93 percent of the population. Reports of illness associated with raw milk (generally cow milk) haven't increased; safety education for farmers may have made a difference. Camels are cleaner and somewhat more disease-resistant than cows. So it's time to legalize some interstate raw milk sales, starting with camel milk, as it's the least allergenic and likely the safest. Creating a structure for interstate raw milk commerce will benefit camel milk customers and expand the market safely.

Researchers are also exploring how the unique attributes of camels might benefit human health. These projects include treatments for seasonal allergies, snakebite, and sexually transmitted diseases. Of course, rigorous scientific studies are needed to understand and prove health benefits. The double-blind, placebo-controlled clinical trial remains the gold standard for evidence. But science can be quite industrialized, and clinical trials, in particular, are generally driven by industry funding. So far, there haven't been sufficient financial incentives for companies to expand the science behind the benefits of camel milk or to package those benefits in a food supplement or drug.

Science tells us what to eat and what to believe about health, but the messages may reflect commercial or political motives. We know that the food industry has influenced US government recommendations on nutrition — like the now-discredited "food pyramid," with its emphasis on carbohydrates — and government agriculture subsidies have led to an abundance of cheap foods that can be detrimental to health. But healthy foods without corporate champions have a hard time attracting attention or financial support. Yet the health and policy issues camel milk raises are relevant even for those who don't need it.

The emphasis on clinical studies and industry funding in science has tended to exclude traditional knowledge, ignoring the voices of people outside the scientific mainstream that could lead to new insights. Science affects everyone's lives, but it remains a highly exclusive club. If you are poor, nonwhite, non-Western, female, or not formally educated, your knowledge and experience are often dismissed as irrelevant. I speak at science conferences, but I'm familiar with that language. Nomads, who have been tending camels and drinking their milk for millennia, are not likely to inspire American science, although studies in camel-producing countries have incorporated nomads' milk and investigated their practices. Health practices whose efficacy has not yet been proved in a clinical trial are mockingly called "woo." But the very word *drug* came from the French for dried herbs, the stuff of traditional medicine. Plants, animals, marine life, and minerals are the sources of our pharmacopeia.

Yet science is gradually recognizing that traditional peoples do hold keys to invaluable knowledge. A relatively new discipline, ethnopharmacology, studies traditional medicines. For example, people in the Boho Highlands of Northern Ireland had long used dirt from a field to treat disease. The soil turned out to contain bacteria that combat antibiotic-resistant superbugs like MRSA. A report by environmental scientists at Yale University acknowledges that indigenous peoples hold wisdom that can contribute to modern science, and the World Bank says that despite their small numbers (4 to 5 percent of the world's population), these peoples live in regions that contain the majority of our planet's biodiversity.

My family is not nomadic, but it has its own forms of traditional knowledge. I was once perplexed about how to transport a carton of fresh cow milk for three hours without a cooler. "I'll have to throw it away," I said.

"Lord, no, honey," said my grandmother. "Ain't you got ye some newspaper?" She wrapped several sheets of newsprint around the carton, which kept it cold for the entire journey. But today's science would tell me to throw it out.

Ironically, even as we're discovering the modern-day uses of camels and their milk, industrialization is encroaching on and destroying their terrain. Plastics litter some deserts, harming camels that eat them. At the site of the Pushkar Fair, helicopter landing pads have been built on the soft dirt where camels used to rest. I saw images of camels with their loyal knees pressed into the rocky surface as the Raika people stood by in frustrated agony. Drones flying overhead at the fair upset both camels and humans. In today's world, nomads are increasingly treated like pieces on a game board, moved around by rolls of the political dice. If a business or government wants more land, nomads are often the first to lose out. But there's good reason to change this.

Climate change hurts the world's most vulnerable people the most. In many parts of the world, nomadic lands are becoming uninhabitable as temperatures in arid regions climb and water dries up. Already many pastoralists are walking much farther to get water for themselves and their animals. The stress caused by shrinking territories and resources leads to clashes between nomadic groups.

But camels are the perfect animals for increasingly parched "dryland" regions in Pakistan, India, Africa, and the Middle East. While they give less milk than cows, it takes far less water and feed to raise them. And people in the Middle East are showing a hearty appetite for camel meat, so nothing of the species would be wasted.

Land and animal stewards like the Amish and nomadic peoples

are undervalued. According to the United Nations assistant secretary general Ibrahim Thiaw, pastoralism should no longer be perceived as "primitive," as he says it's not an unproductive, antienvironmental occupation, as some myths hold.

Milk and meat from pastoralists provide food security and valued nutrients to local populations, says Bernard Faye, a camel expert with the UN's Food and Agriculture Organization. And technology can assist. In Ethiopia, satellite imagery is being used to identify good grazing areas, which are divided to minimize clashes between herder clans. This supports herder coexistence and has led to a 47 percent reduction in livestock deaths.

Still, one way or another, most of the world's nomadic camel-herding peoples are being driven from their land. Economic and political challenges lead them to quit the nomadic lifestyle and move to the city, as the Raika youth are doing, or move to a foreign country and send money home, like my friend Sidi Amar, a Tuareg from Niger who trains American camels. (Sidi, who had no shoes until age sixteen, says a nomadic lifestyle is the healthiest and best, and this is borne out by a study of children in northern Kenya.) These pressures can have particularly severe consequences for girls and women, whose education and well-being are often the first to be sacrificed in times of hardship (pastoral women traditionally sell milk and manage the proceeds). Money-strapped families in camel countries may lose their daughters to child marriage, trafficking, or infanticide.

All these problems are heavy straws to place on a camel's back. But a thriving camel industry could unite agribusiness interests, farmers and landholders, health providers, climate professionals, women's advocates, and upholders of tribal cultures. A camel milk industry offers a chance for increased income, health, and peace.

There are successful models for camel keepers to follow. Gil and Nancy at Oasis Camel Dairy in California now have a satisfying home-based business. They finally bought the adjoining farm they'd been eyeing for years. It holds a warehouse of imported Al Nassma camel milk chocolate, made from Camelicious milk. They've fixed up the farmhouse as a vacation rental, so that visitors can wake up and watch the camel herd stroll, play, and run. They've even pioneered a new, gentle form of camel training, based on rewards and the camel's natural desires.

In India, Dr. Ilse Köhler-Rollefson has started the Kumbhalgarh Camel Dairy, selling Raika herders' milk. Ilse says their dairy pays the herders more than would-be competitors. In a video chat with Magan Raika at the dairy's grand opening, musicians played for me as a circle of herders smiled and said, "Namaste." "We need you here," he said, bringing tears to my eyes.

In America, more merchants are making camel milk soap, lotion, and beauty products, including lipstick. And powdered camel milk from other countries is now approved for sale. Some US farmers still sell milk to Walid's distribution company. He offers a low price, but they see little alternative at present. Yet demand for the milk is rising as the secret slowly gets out. The farmers' herds are small but growing.

All in all, camels are more popular than ever. They're being used for food, rides, therapy, weddings, advertisements, and television — even as a motif in interior decoration. All this positive exposure is good for camels around the world. Society fails animals that no one knows exist. And, as I saw in India, an animal without purpose becomes a living fossil.

These new developments make one thing clear. The camel is still indispensable, a loyal and valued livestock animal and companion. The days of camel darkness should end here and now. It's time to "look at the camel," as the Qur'an says, and welcome it into our lives.

APPENDIX

Camel Milk: A Users' Guide

USES OF CAMEL MILK

Camel milk has been used for centuries as a healing substance and highly nutritious food. It is high in vitamins and contains immunoglobulins, enzymes, and many other ingredients that can boost immune system function, combat bacteria and other germs, and enhance healing.

Camel milk may be beneficial in treating conditions associated with inflammation, which may include:

- autism spectrum disorder (ASD)
- attention deficit disorder (ADD), attention deficit hyperactivity disorder (ADHD)
- gastrointestinal problems: irritable bowel disease, Crohn's disease, diarrhea, loose stools
- diabetes
- skin conditions such as eczema and psoriasis
- failure to thrive
- food allergy, intolerance, and sensitivity
- Hashimoto's thyroiditis
- sugar sensitivity

- yeast overgrowth or thrush
- chemotherapy-induced fatigue, anemia, mouth sores, and other side effects
- Machado-Joseph disease
- kidney damage
- rheumatoid arthritis
- liver damage
- sensory dysfunction

PROPERTIES OF CAMEL MILK
Nutritional Profile

This table presents a nutritional analysis of eight ounces of frozen raw American camel milk (a blend of milk from ten camels, supplied by Marlin Troyer) by an independent laboratory.

Nutritional Analysis of 8 Ounces of Frozen Raw American Camel Milk

Calories	107.360 kcal
Protein	5.392 g
Sugar	8.296 g
Carbohydrate	10.956 g
Fat	4.0–4.6 g
Vitamin A	224.480 IU
Iron	0.395 mg
Calcium	292.800 mg

Vitamin Concentration

Vitamin Concentration of Various Mammalian Milks

	Goat (in 100 g)	Sheep (in 100 g)	Cattle (in 100 g)	Human (in 100 g)	Camel (in 100 mL)[†]
Vitamin A (IU), (*μg)	185	146	126	190	26.7*
Vitamin D (IU), (*μg)	2.3	1.18*	2	1.4	0.3*
Thiamin (mg)	0.068	0.08	0.045	0.017	0.048
Riboflavin (mg)	0.21	0.376	0.16	0.02	0.168
Niacin (mg)	0.27	0.416	0.08	0.17	0.77
Pantothenic acid (mg)	0.31	0.408	0.32	0.2	0.368
Vitamin B6 (mg)	0.046	0.08	0.042	0.011	0.55
Folic acid (μg)	1	5	5	5.5	87
Biotin (μg)	1.5	0.93	2	0.4	–
Vitamin B12 (μg)	0.065	0.712	0.357	0.03	85
Vitamin C (mg)	1.29	4.16	0.94	5	33

[†] *For liquids of this approximate density, 100 g is essentially the same amount as 100 mL.*

Source: J. Barłowska, M. Szwajkowska, Z. Litwińczuk, and J. Król, "Nutritional Value and Technological Suitability of Milk from Various Animal Species Used for Dairy Production," *Comprehensive Reviews in Food Science and Food Safety* 10, no. 6 (November 2011): 291–302, https://onlinelibrary.wiley.com/doi/full/10.1111/j.1541-4337.2011.00163.x.

Composition

Composit on of Milk of Mammals (g/10 mL)

	Human	Cow	Buffalo	Goat	Sheep	Camel	Mare	Donkey
Fat	3.6	3.9	6.6	3.8	7.3	4.9	2.1	2.0
Protein	1.2	3.3	0.6	3.9	5.7	3.5	1.7	1.5
Lactose	6.4	4.3	4.7	4.7	4.6	5.0	6.2	6.3
Minerals	0.2	0.6	0.7	0.8	0.8	0.8	0.5	0.4
Water	88.6	87.9	87.4	86.8	81.6	85.8	89.5	89.8
pH	7.1	6.5	6.7	6.5	6.5	6.5	6.7	7.1
SG (specific gravity)	1.03	1.03	1.03	1.03	1.03	1.03	1.03	1.03
Calories	63	66	81	69	107	78	50	49

Source: M. O. Swar, "Donkey Milk-Based Formula: A Substitute for Patients with Cow's Milk Protein Allergy," *Sudanese Journal of Paediatrics* 11, no. 2 (2011): 21–24, https://www.ncbi.nlm.nih.gov/pmc/articles/PMC4949830/.

Taste

The first thing people ask about camel milk is, "What does it taste like?" Once they try it, they usually say, "It tastes just like milk!" That's because it *is* milk. In some countries, and depending on the camels' diet, people report a slight salty taste, but in camel milk from the United States this flavor is not pronounced.

After you've been drinking it for a while, you'll notice that milks from different sources have slightly different flavors. You'll learn to appreciate them in the same way that people enjoy fine cheeses.

BUYING AND HANDLING CAMEL MILK
Raw, Pasteurized, or Powdered?

Raw camel milk is the most effective form, because pasteurization may destroy some potentially beneficial compounds. However, raw milk may be difficult to obtain. Freeze-dried, spray-dried, or flash-pasteurized milk (which is heated and held at 161.6°F or 72°C for only 15–18 seconds) can also be effective for treating various conditions and has excellent nutritional value. If pasteurized camel milk does not seem effective, it may be worth trying to locate a safe source of raw milk.

If liquid milk is hard to find, powdered camel milk is available in single-serving packages in Europe, the Middle East, and India, and in larger sealed packages in the United States and other places. Powdered milk comes in two forms: spray-dried and freeze-dried. Freeze-dried milk is thought to retain more beneficial components (such as immunoglobulins) than spray-dried. Powdered milk comes in white or slightly yellow flakes and may have a more pronounced taste than liquid milk. It can be reconstituted with water according to package directions or simply stirred into moist foods or liquids.

Safety

Raw camel milk should be sourced only from herds regularly tested for diseases that can affect humans, such as brucellosis and tuberculosis. (American camels do not have the disease MERS [Middle Eastern respiratory syndrome] that affects some herds in other countries.) To ensure safety, ask to see official lab results, veterinary records, and milk batch tests. The supplier should keep a record of the lots it sells; you can keep records of your purchases too.

Hygienic handling, storage, and shipping processes are also vital to ensure the safety of milk. Most US suppliers observe state standards for testing and hygiene.

Pasteurizing Milk at Home

Pasteurizing raw milk at home is simple to do and may be the best choice if you have any doubts about the safety or quality of your supply.

The method below is supplied by Nancy Abeiderrahmane, founder of the Tiviski Camel Dairy and a pioneer in the making of camel cheese.

Use a medium saucepan and a home cooking thermometer. Do not preheat the pan, as this may scorch the milk and create an unpleasant taste.

Heat the milk in the pan, testing it with the thermometer intermittently. Once the temperature reaches 161.6°F (72°C), quickly remove the pan from the heat, wait 15–18 seconds (measured by the clock), and then pour the milk into a heat-resistant bottle or container, such as a glass or stainless-steel jar. Immerse the container in ice water for fast chilling. Store the milk in a refrigerator in a closed container. It will keep for eight to fifteen days.

The first attempt can be tricky, as the milk appears to heat slowly but comes to temperature rather quickly. A wrinkled skin may appear on the surface of the milk if it overheats. But practice will make you an expert in no time.

Thawing and Storing

Fresh camel milk should be stored in the refrigerator. According to standard US guidelines, it's best drunk within five to seven days.

However, many consumers drink milk up to fourteen days old; some like the tangy taste that develops and believe that the bacteria responsible for the taste are beneficial.

Frozen camel milk can be thawed by placing the bottle in cool water in a sink or countertop bowl for two to three hours. Set a timer as a reminder to remove and refrigerate the bottle.

Powdered camel milk can be stored for up to a year in a cool, dry place such as a pantry. After that it can grow a bit sour.

Some people ask whether they can thaw frozen milk, place it in smaller containers, and refreeze it. I feel this may somewhat damage beneficial compounds in the milk, but many users report no concerns. Although refreezing completely thawed foods may pose health risks, the federal government considers refreezing milk to be safe if the milk is still slushy and contains ice crystals or has been at a temperature over 40°F for no more than two hours. You may experience a loss of texture and quality, but the milk is still a good source of nutrition and likely beneficial. Small milk suppliers may be willing to provide you with milk in smaller containers (possibly at an additional cost). It's also possible to cut a plastic bottle in half with a bread knife (be careful!) and thaw half at a time.

Traveling with Camel Milk

When traveling with fresh or frozen camel milk, pack it in an insulated cooler with plenty of freezer packs. If you're taking it as carry-on luggage on a flight, bring a doctor's letter documenting your need for it to get through security. If you're packing it in checked luggage, wrap the milk bottles in newsprint, pack them tightly together, and enclose with freezer packs in a Styrofoam-type or insulated container.

For international travel, check the biosecurity regulations governing the importation of dairy products in the destination country. You may need to supply a doctor's letter documenting a medical need, and you might also consider packing a nutrition label from the supplier.

USING CAMEL MILK
How Much?

If you are healthy and are interested in camel milk for enhancing over-all wellness or because you're at risk for a particular health condition, you can drink as much or as little as you want.

For people with specific health conditions, the amount consumed should be measured and monitored until you have determined an amount that's effective and causes no adverse effects. There is no set amount that's right for every person or every condition. You'll learn what works through trial and observation.

Start with the smallest amount indicated in the table below and in-crease by one-half ounce to one ounce every other day as the body adjusts. If this amount is well tolerated, with no or minor side effects, increase it by one ounce per day to suit personal preferences and needs. If side effects occur, decrease by one-half ounce to one ounce per day until the body adjusts, then try increasing the amount again.

Reports indicate that drinking more than two cups per day does not increase effectiveness for most known conditions. However, children and people with limited choices of safe food sources often drink more with no problems.

Below are suggested daily servings for different child age groups and for adults with different conditions. (All numbers in these tables are approximate and rounded off for conversion from ounces to milli-liters.) These should be adjusted for the individual's situation. Guide-lines for nursing mothers are given in a separate section below.

Suggested Daily Camel-Milk Servings for Children

Age	Amount
6 months–2 years	½ oz (15 mL), working up to 4 oz (120 mL)
2–6 years	2–4 oz (60–120 mL)
7–10 years	3–4 oz (90–120 mL)
11–17 years	3–6 oz (90–180 mL)

NOTE: Adjust the amount of milk according to the size and weight of the child as well as age. If a child is very sensitive to foods, start with ¼ to ½ teaspoon of milk and increase to the recommended amount as tolerated or needed. Milk can be given every other day rather than daily if no regression or symptom reappearance occurs. Additional milk can be given as needed for specific uses like dietary infractions (such as ingesting cow milk or gluten when on the casein-free and gluten-free diet) or if sugar, carbohydrates, or other foods cause hyperactivity, rashes, or gastrointestinal symptoms.

Suggested Daily Camel-Milk Servings for Adults with Different Conditions

Condition	Amount	Notes
General supplement or preventative	4 oz (120 mL)	
Crohn's disease	1 cup / 8 oz+ (240 mL+)	
Juvenile rheumatoid arthritis	4 oz+ (120 mL+)	
Chronic inflammation	4 oz+ (120 mL+)	
Diabetes (types 1 and 2)	4–17 oz (120–500 mL) (In most diabetes studies, the recommended dose of camel milk was 500 mL/day, which led to improvement of diabetes markers.)	Adjust insulin dose to account for the milk's nutritional content (protein, fat, etc.) and test blood sugar before and after drinking.
Machado-Joseph disease	16 oz (480 mL)	
Chemo recovery	8–16 oz (240–480 mL)	May reduce mouth sores and inflammation and aid recovery between chemo rounds.

NOTE: Milk can be consumed every other day or at longer intervals in some conditions, as long as symptoms are controlled. Keep a journal of symptoms and milk serving size and frequency, then see how symptoms compare to lab-obtained medical markers from a doctor. This can provide data on the milk's usefulness.

How Long Will It Take to Work?

Some users show a positive response within eight hours. For others, it may take two to three months for systemic benefits to become evident. Raw milk often produces faster and more dramatic results. The milk may not produce improvements in everyone.

Possible Side Effects

Camel milk occasionally produces mild adverse symptoms in some people. Reported side effects include irritability, hyperactivity, disrupted sleep, more talking or babbling, loose or discolored stools, skin flushing, and mild tics. These typically diminish over time and disappear if the amount of milk is reduced. If disrupted sleep is a problem, try serving the milk early in the day.

Some of these effects may come from the milk's ability to kill pathogens: as the pathogens die off, toxins are released from their cells. This is known as the die-off or Jarisch-Herxheimer response, and it is also occasionally seen with some antibiotics and antifungal treatments. In addition, reduction of inflammation and autism symptoms may reveal underlying problems that were previously masked (such as intermittent tic disorder).

Do I Have to Use It Forever?

How long to continue using camel milk depends on the individual's response to it. I believe most users with ASD that is affected by diet can benefit from remaining on the milk. But the expense can make that difficult. In some children with autism spectrum disorders, symptoms may improve as they mature, and use of camel milk can be reduced.

Some adults with severe gastrointestinal issues, immune system disorders, food intolerance, or rheumatoid arthritis report that they need to keep drinking the milk to manage their condition. Adults with diabetes may experience increased blood-sugar control with continued consumption of camel milk and any needed medication, although some with type 2 diabetes may be able to discontinue medication by following an appropriate diet (which may include camel milk).

Some people with food allergy and intolerance who try camel milk continue to show significant improvement after discontinuing consumption. The decision to stop camel milk can be made in consultation with an informed doctor or allergist who has read the scientific literature on camel milk, or users can read this themselves. There are anecdotal reports of Machado-Joseph syndrome symptoms returning when camel milk intake is lowered.

Using Camel Milk to Reduce ASD Symptoms

Camel milk can be effective in reducing autism symptoms in some children. It's best used in conjunction with other dietary and therapeutic interventions. But aggression and other symptoms of autism may worsen as puberty hits or other changes occur. Judicious use of medications is sometimes necessary to manage aggression and agitation. Doctors specializing in autism, such as neurologists and psychiatrists, can prescribe such medications.

Preparing to Introduce Camel Milk

The most effective dietary intervention for ASD is to remove all dairy products from the child's diet. This includes products made from cow, goat, or sheep, such as whey, butter, casein, and milk powder. I recommend removing all soy, nut, and rice milks as well. Lowering intake of refined carbohydrates and sugars and increasing proteins and vegetables is beneficial for many and aligns with basic health guidelines. I also recommend an organic diet. Some children and adults benefit from removal of gluten, a protein found in wheat and other food products.

If it's not possible to stop consumption of all dairy products because of nutritional needs or other constraints, one approach is to gradually replace them with camel milk. For example, you can reduce the consumption of cow milk by one ounce (30 mL) each day and replace it with the same amount of camel milk. This lessens the chance of rejection, but it does make it more difficult to judge the effectiveness of camel milk and may diminish its benefits until the transition is complete.

Before starting camel milk, observe the child's behavior and document it with photos and videos to provide a baseline for assessing changes. Gather records of blood work and other medical history, as well as school reports.

Testing for Tolerance

Although allergic reactions to camel milk are exceedingly rare, it's wise to eliminate the possibility before you introduce the milk into your child's diet. For kids with known allergies and severe food intolerances, tests should be conducted under the care of a doctor, preferably an allergist. Be sure to have a rescue treatment on hand. But for those who aren't highly reactive to allergens, you can try this yourself. Choose a time when you can observe the child continuously. Soak a cotton ball in camel milk and tape it to the skin with a bandage or medical tape (typical places are the inner arm above the elbow or the back). Leave the ball in place for a reasonable length of time. Some leave it for only an hour, others for up to twenty-four hours. If redness, burning, or itching occurs at any time, remove and wash the skin immediately. If you see nothing, proceed.

Introducing Camel Milk

You can start a child on camel milk at any time of the day. Some parents prefer to give it on an empty stomach for a faster effect, but it can also be accompanied by a light meal or snack, particularly if you see extreme hyperactivity or irritability.

Sleep may either improve or be disrupted at first. If mild adverse responses occur initially, reduce the amount of camel milk. You may also want to try a different brand of milk, since its composition can vary depending on the animals' diet, lactation stage, and other factors, and even minute amounts of allergens from a specific farm environment can cause an allergic response.

Adjusting Amount for Age, Size, and Individual Situation

Adjust the recommended amount in the table above according to the child's size. Weight variances are common among kids with autism.

Some are underweight from feeding issues and malabsorption of nutrients; others may be overweight from gut disturbances, medications, inactivity, and food-seeking behavior.

Some picky eaters and kids who are failing to thrive will gain weight on camel milk. Some heavier kids may slim down, because the milk, in conjunction with a healthy diet, may help appease hunger and stabilize blood sugar levels.

If your child occasionally eats foods that trigger negative autism-related behaviors and other symptoms (aggression, emotional upset, rigidity, perseverations, stimming [self-stimulatory behavior, such as repetitive movement or speech], rashes, bowel problems), camel milk may alleviate them, sometimes in as little as twenty minutes.

Observing

While using camel milk, keep a journal or log noting the child's feelings, language, and levels of functioning. Take photos and videos of the child's behavior. Adults may keep a record of their own reactions. Request new medical tests to assess physiological changes.

Making Camel Milk Appealing to Children

Since many children are sensitive to taste or fanciful of mind, don't tell them that the milk comes from camels (unless you know they won't care). The easiest way to start is by substituting it for the milk you are currently using (either dairy or nondairy).

Chocolate and other syrups can be mixed with the milk. Smoothies and milkshakes are popular with kids and have the added advantage that they can be served in a cup with a lid to conceal them (some autistic kids can detecting the slightest difference in food's smell or appearance). Either follow the smoothie recipe below or blend some dairy-free ice cream with camel milk, add a wide straw, and offer with a minimum of fanfare. (Don't act too enthusiastic, or they may suspect something different.)

Some handy parents make yogurt, but making yogurt with camel milk can be more challenging than using cow or goat milk because different yogurt cultures are needed and camel milk does not coagulate in the same way (the product will be runny).

For children who refuse all drinks other than water (there are some), you can try offering the milk in a squirt-style syringe, using food or toys as behavioral reinforcement. If they reject the milk, don't force them. Slowly add it to foods like warm macaroni and dairy-free cheese (stir it in, unheated, just before serving), pour it on cereal, oatmeal, pancakes, or cake, dunk cookies in it, or soak a fruit popsicle in it. For very difficult cases, engage an occupational or eating therapist, and be patient.

CAMEL MILK SMOOTHIE RECIPE

This basic recipe is suitable for a child or adult. It makes a mildly flavored sweet drink (use more fruit juice to add zing). Agave nectar is a low-glycemic-index sweetener, meaning that it is absorbed more slowly by the body than cane sugar. Coconut water contains potassium and has approximately half the sugars of fruit juice.

The recipe can be easily doubled. A teaspoon of date sugar is a nice sub-stitute for the agave, as it contains fiber and potassium and is made of dried dates (traditionally often served with camel milk). Date sugar pairs well with banana and pineapple fruit. Honey may also be used instead of agave, but it tends to form clumps. Some nutritionists recommend using low-acid fruits with camel milk (lists can be found online). Powdered dietary supplements can be added if desired, but additional liquid and fruit may be needed for ease of blending and to mask the taste. Some powdered dietary supplements can be beneficial for children with autism, if your autism practitioner approves.

½ cup (4 ounces / 120 mL) liquid camel milk or reconstituted
     powdered camel milk
1 cup (8 ounces / 240 mL) frozen fruit
¼ cup (2 ounces / 60 mL) coconut water
¼ cup (2 ounces / 60 mL) fruit juice or premade bottled smoothie
1 teaspoon (5 mL) agave nectar, or more to taste

Place all ingredients in a blender jar. Blend for 5–10 seconds. Serve immediately.

Camel Milk for Nursing Mothers

Nursing mothers may be advised by their doctors to remove potential or known allergens from their own diets, as they can pass these to babies through breast milk. Removing dairy products (cow or goat milk, whey, yogurt, cheese, and butter) from the mother's diet and replacing them with camel milk may prevent some infants' reactions to dairy products and improve their food tolerance while providing a good source of calcium and other nutrients. Nursing mothers should consult a lactation expert or doctor to ensure appropriate nutrition.

WHERE TO BUY CAMEL MILK

In most countries, consumers can now purchase camel milk through local farms and herders or online suppliers. In addition to the sources listed, there may be small farms or other providers in your area, so ask camel owners or grocery store managers for recommendations. Not all the suppliers listed here have postal addresses, phone numbers, or websites. The listings may change at any time.

Laws and practices governing the purchase of raw milk vary by state and country. This list is not intended as a guarantee of safety or quality. Ask providers for current herd health certificates / vet tests and milk safety tests. In countries where camels are common, you might also contact the animal science department of a local university.

US Distributors

DESERT FARMS USA
*products are available online
and at stores nationwide*
Walid Abdul-Wahab
2708 Wilshire Blvd. #380
Santa Monica, CA 90403
Phone: 800-430-7426
camelmilk@desertfarms.com
www.desertfarms.com

CAMEL MILK COOPERATIVE
products available online
142 North Street
Ridgefield, CT 06877
Phone: 561-236-8008
info@camelmilkcoop.com
www.camelmilkcoop.com

CAMILK DAIRY
products available online
info@camilkdairy.com
www.camilkdairy.com

DROMEDAIRY NATURALS USA
camel milk powder available online
Michael Cassio, CEO
7200 S. Alton Way A340
Centennial, CO 80112
Phone: 303-717-0379
sales@dromedairy.com
www.dromedairy.us

SAHARA DAIRY COMPANY
products available online
Bryce Hallam
4695 MacArthur Court,
11th Floor
Newport Beach, CA 92660
Phone: 530-318-0113
info@saharadairyco.com
www.saharadairyco.com

THE CAMEL MILK CO.
*products available online and
at retail locations*
Ryan Fee
17032 Campo Drive
Parker, CO 80134
Phone: 720-515-4746
sales@thecamelmilkco.com
www.thecamelmilkco.com

US Farmers

CAMEL MILK ASSOCIATION
Marlin Troyer
8380 S. Tyndall Road
Branch, MI 49402
Phone: 231-878-6528
info@camelmilkassociation.org
www.camelmilkassociation.org

CAMELOT CAMEL DAIRY LLC
Kyle and Holly Hendrix
50643 CR KK
Wray, CO 80758
Phone: 970-630-2761
camelotcameldairy@gmail.com
www.camelotcameldairy.com

COLORADO CAMEL MILK
Joseph and Nicole Henderson
15493 North 107th Street
Longmont, CO 80504
Phone: 720-232-7030
nbell_98@yahoo.com
www.coloradocamelmilk.com

DROME-DAIRY
Noah Peachey
16073 State Route 405
Watsontown, PA 17777
Phone: 570-538-1302

HUMPBACK DAIRY
Sam and Jeff Hostetler
4858 Lawrence 1185
Miller, MO 65707
Phone: 417-848-7570

MILLER'S ORGANIC FARM
648 Millcreek School Road
Bird-in-Hand, PA 17505
Phone: 717-556-0672
www.millersorganicfarm.com

International Sources

Australia

AUSTRALIA CAMEL MILK NSW
1618 Denman Road
Muswellbrook, NSW 2333
Phone: +61 0408 677 741
info@camelmilknsw.com.au
www.camelmilknsw.com.au

CALAMUNNDA CAMEL FARM
Chris O'Hora
361 Paulls Valley Road
Kalamunda, WA 6076
Phone: +61 8 9293 1156
camelbooking@gmail.com
www.camelfarm.com

CAMILK PTY LTD
156 Morton Road
Rochester, VIC 3561
Phone: +61 3 5484 1623
info@camilkdairy.com
www.camilkdairy.com

Q CAMEL DAIRY
Lauren Brisbane, Director
165 Sahara Road
Glasshouse Mountains,
QLD 4518
Phone: +61 7 5438 7890
sales@qcamel.com.au
www.qcamel.com.au

THE AUSTRALIAN WILD CAMEL
CORPORATION (SUMMER LAND)
8 Charles Chauvel Drive
Harrisville, QLD 4307
Phone: +61 7 5467 1707
admin@summerlandcamels
.com.au
www.summerlandcamels.com.au

THE CAMEL MILK CO
Tee Rowe
Kyabram, VIC 3620
Phone: +61 4 1753 3733
sales@camelmilkco.com.au
www.camelmilkco.com.au

Egypt

TAYYIBA FARMS
Phone: +20 02 01555678 777
inquires@tayyibafarms.com
www.tayyibafarms.com

Germany

KAMELFARM MARQUARD
Hiddinger Str. 48
27374 Visselhovede
Hiddingen
Phone: +49 171-9840576
info@kamelfarm.de
www.kamelfarm.de

India

AADVIK FOODS
Hitesh Rathi, CEO
Phone: +91 8800638181
info@aadvikfoods.com
www.aadvikfoods.com

CAMEL CHARISMA
Dr. Ilse Köhler-Rollefson,
Hanwant Singh Rathore
Butibagh, Rajpura
Sadri 306702, District Pali,
Rajasthan
Phone: +91 9660083437
info@camelcharisma.com
www.camelcharisma.com

SHE-CAMEL
Kahkashan Quraishi
Langer Toli, Bari Path, near
Goodman Publication
Patna, Bihar
Phone: +91 8809474694
fquraishi412@gmail.com
www.she-camel.com

Israel

CAMELAND NEGEV CAMEL
RANCH
Phone: +972 8 6552829
kurnob@gmail.com
www.cameland.co.il

Kazakhstan

DAULET-BEKET FARM
27 Konayeva Street
Village of Aisha, Ily Borough,
Almaty region
Phone: +7 727 393-44-95;
+7 701 777-91-20
Fax: +7 727 300-12-18
daulet-beket@mail.run

Kenya

WHITE GOLD CAMEL MILK
Jama Warsame, CEO
Ngamia Milk Suppliers
Phone: +254 791 801243
PO Box 175
Nanyuki 10400
jwarsame1976@gmail.com
www.whitegoldcamelmilk.com

SPIERS LTD
Piers Simpkin, CEO
PO Box 379
Nairobi 00502
Phone: +44 723950360
spiersent06@yahoo.co.uk

Malaysia

CAMELAIT CAMEL MILK ASIA
Shah Alam
www.camelait.asia/where-to
-buy

Mauritania

TIVISKI CAMEL DAIRY
Nagi Ichidou, CEO
B.P. 2069, Nouakchott
nagi@tiviski.com
www.tiviski.com

Morocco

LAIT DE CHAMELLE
Abdul, salesperson
Risanni
Phone: +212 6 3907 4860

Netherlands

CAMEL PRODUCTS
sales@camelproducts.eu
www.camelproducts.eu

KAMELENMELKERIJ SMITS
Frank Smits
frank@kamelenmelk.nl
www.kamelenmelk.nl

South Africa

CAMEL MILK SOUTH AFRICA
39 Helderzicht Road
Somerset West 7130
Phone: +972 81 043 9621; +972
73 377 1567; +972 83 272 2164
admin@camelmilksouthafrica
.co.za
camelmilksouthafrica.co.za
/products/fresh-milk

United Arab Emirates

CAMELAIT
Al Ain Farms
PO Box 15571, Al Foah
Al Ain, Abu Dhabi
Phone: +971 37114600
info@camelait.net
www.camelait.net

CAMELICIOUS
Emirates Industry for Camel
Milk and Products
Al Ain Road, Exit 26
Umm Nahad 3, Dubai
Phone: +971 42281034
Fax: +971 42281039
info@camelicious.ae
www.camelicious.ae

United Kingdom

DESERT FARMS UK AND EU
Phone: +44 203 695 8445
camelmilk@desertfarms.co.uk
www.desertfarms.co.uk

HUMP GROUP
Unit 002F, IBIC 2, Holt Court
South, Birmingham Science Park
Aston
Holt Street
Birmingham, West Midlands,
B7 4EJ
Phone: +44 755 443 4426
hello@humpgroup.co.uk
www.humpgroup.co.uk

ACKNOWLEDGMENTS

Since I first met the camel that sent me on a quest, I've come to know some highly interesting people. I've relied on a chain of helpers and experts that now extends around the world. We worked together to make this book and I am proud they wanted to be in it. Communicating about camels is not the easiest thing. It involves opposite time zones, remote locations, language barriers, and trusting the faces you've seen only in pictures. All these twists and turns just made the experience more fun.

But as with every endeavor, the journey starts at home. The people closest to me have been the most amazing.

My beautiful stepdaughters, Gwen, Juli, and Christina, mean so much to me. Together we've made memories, opened joke presents, eaten their dad's bounteous dinners, auditioned boyfriends, and made a family. They accepted Jonah and me into their lives and shared their father with us. They are brave, nonjudgmental, nonmaterialistic, and smart. And thanks to my son-in-law Harold, who makes me the best ice cream.

There is too much to say about my son, Jonah. But whatever there is to say, he will always say it best. He's a savvy and insightful young man. Talented, witty, verbally gifted, he makes me laugh. He's kind, polite, empathetic, and industrious. We have gone through so much together; no one but us could understand it. Our bond is ever strong, our love unbreakable.

My husband Tony's goodness shines through to everyone in his life. He has so many skills and gifts, but never judges those who don't, and uplifts them instead. It's incredible that I found him in this fast-paced day and age. He led my heart to a happier place by nurturing my son and me. Despite the demands of his own busy life, he's my most thoughtful reader and supporter. The book is both of ours, thanks to the years of loving, patient effort he put into supporting it and me. I love him beyond words.

I appreciate my sisters, Trish and Dana. People admire and depend on them. Their hospitality to me and mine is forever cherished. And the world needs more sincere and intelligent young men like my nephews Andrew and Justin.

No one could ever have raised a kid like me as well as my mother, Gail, did. She gave me Southern mountain values along with the intellectual freedom to read, speak, and do as I wished (most of the time). We've come a long way for a coal miner's daughter and granddaughter. Her own intelligence and never-ending curiosity for books and the natural world illuminated my path.

My aunts, uncles, and cousins are a wonderful bunch of folks. They work hard, believe in good, and give their best effort to everything they do. I miss my late father and my relatives, with their understated Appalachian strength and humor. They were role models for kindness and bearing hardships with dignity.

The cameleers who populate this book have been generous with their time, camels, and deeds. I appreciate their honesty, passion, and willingness to help others.

Camel veterinarians and scientists offered me courtesy and were very inclusive and welcoming. They're kind, inquisitive, smart, and essential friends to camels.

Some doctors I connected with applied their own valuable insights to my topic. This is medicine as it should be: open-minded, incisive, and scientifically critical. Dr. Caroline Choan, Dr. Robin Eckert,

Dr. Koren Barrett, Dr. Amnon Gonenne, Dr. David Riley, Dr. Doreen Granpeesheh, and Dr. Deeba Baig are greatly appreciated.

Writers can't make it without other writers' support. They connect you to others and lend perceptive eyes and ears. I thank Barbara Demarco Barrett, Anita Hughes, Caroline Leavitt, Madhushree Ghosh, Jimin Han, Martin Smith, Joann Mapson, Kathryn Abajian, the Binders, and many more. And Joel Salatin fit me into his crazy schedule and honored the book with his moving and expressive foreword.

And without an agent, a book can go nowhere. Dana Newman is resourceful, deft, and patient and gets complex concepts easily, a rare and wonderful ability. The perfect publisher emerged for me: the fabulous New World Library. Editor Georgia Hughes is deeply perceptive, enthusiastic, and wonderful to work with. I thank her, Monique Muhlenkamp, and the rest of the NWL team for their excitement and commitment.

Helping friends Guadalupe Valente, Bash Kazi, Yasser Barakat, Martin Lilley, Rohini Bedi, Parvis Zarinpour, Shannon Penrod, Sidi Amar, Guy Seeklus, Tayla Hart, Pete Kennedy, Vanessa Bull, Kristen Clarfeld, Manish Sharma, Michelle Mittleman, Loupa Pius Da, Cara Burns, Randi Winter, and so many others provided something special to this journey.

The health and autism communities reveal the greatest strength. They work their way through a landscape of challenges, leading their kids so bravely. And two little brothers named Jethro and Leander Troyer will always be remembered with love.

I deeply thank the pastoral and nomadic people who participated in this book. They want their legacies preserved and their voices expressed. They struggle against obstacles that would make most people despair or quit. But they're out there in the world, doing good things for our planet, yet remaining largely unseen. Their ancestral knowledge, willingness to share, and devotion to animals are beacons of enlightenment.

And I thank the camels, who smile because they know how special they are.

NOTES

INTRODUCTION

p. xvi *estimated at thirty-five million*: "Gateway to Dairy Production and Products: Camels," Food and Agriculture Organization of the United Nations, accessed August 6, 2019, http://www.fao.org/dairy -production-products/production/dairy-animals/camels/en/.

p. xvi *twenty million during my first year of research:* "The Next Thing: Camel Milk," Food and Agriculture Organization of the United Nations, April 18, 2006, http://www.fao.org/newsroom/en/news/2006 /1000275/index.html.

CHAPTER 2. THE NEXT STEP

p. 6 *"Etiology of Autism and Camel Milk as Therapy":* Yosef Shabo et al., "Etiology of Autism and Camel Milk as Therapy," *International Journal on Disability and Human Development*, April 2005, https://www .researchgate.net/publication/276038302_Etiology_of_autism_and _camel_milk_as_therapy.

p. 6 *"Camel Milk for Food Allergies in Children":* Yosef Shabo et al., "Camel Milk for Food Allergies in Children," *Israel Medical Association Journal* 7, no. 12 (Dec. 2005): 796–98, abstract available at https://www.ncbi .nlm.nih.gov/pubmed/16382703.

p. 6 *It makes my son flap his hands:* Emily Delzell, "Idiopathic Toe Walking: Insights on Intervention," LER, August 2012, https://lermagazine .com/article/idiopathic-toe-walking-insights-on-intervention.

CHAPTER 6. AN OASIS OF CAMELS

p. 26 *"The idea of the IUD came from camels":* Sarah Laskow, "The Twisted History of IUD Design," *Atlas Obscura*, May 3, 2017, https://www .atlasobscura.com/articles/iud-design-history-contraception.

CHAPTER 8. THE MILK KNOWS NO BORDERS

p. 38   *"If you think camel milk helps autism, you're stupid":* This doctor did apologize later, but I was ready to move on.

CHAPTER 9. CAMELS: A GOD-GIVEN MARVEL?

p. 40   *they can lose up to 40 percent of their body weight in water:* "Blood Cells Protect from Dehydration," AskNature, September 14, 2016, https://asknature.org/strategy/blood-cells-protect-from-dehydration.

p. 43   *After centuries of ranging freely on this land:* "The Beginning of the End for Israel's Negev Bedouin Culture," The Observers, July 17, 2013, https://observers.france24.com/en/20130717-end-israel-negev-bedouin-culture; Jack Khoury, "Israel Revokes Citizenship of Hundreds of Negev Bedouin, Leaving Them Stateless," *Haaretz*, August 25, 2017, https://www.haaretz.com/israel-news/.premium-israel-revokes-citizenship-of-hundreds-of-bedouin-1.5445620.

p. 43   *"I hope that you can provide me with a scientific answer":* Islam Question & Answer, March 27, 2006, https://islamqa.info/en/answers/83423/the-benefits-of-drinking-camel-urine.

p. 44   *An oral Arab and nomadic Muslim proverb:* I asked many Muslims about this matter. A few imams I consulted said, "The camel is great," but added that this saying isn't Islamic and isn't found in the Qur'an; moreover, they said that the names of Allah are not limited to ninety-nine, and there's no way to know them all.

CHAPTER 11. GETTING CLOSE TO CAMELS

p. 51   *"One night, we found seven camels":* Christina Adams, "The Camel Whisperer of California," OZY, July 15, 2016, https://www.ozy.com/rising-stars/the-camel-whisperer-of-california/70285.

CHAPTER 13. A PUBLIC BIRTH

p. 59   *the article I've been writing for weeks:* See Christina Adams, "Got [Camel] Milk?," *Autism File*, March 12, 2012, 47–50, http://christinaadamsauthor.com/wp-content/uploads/2018/06/AF_43_CamelMilkl.LR_.pdf.

p. 63   *it's based on a variant of* coucher: "Origin and Etymology of Kush/Cush in Regards to Animals," Stack Exchange, February 28, 2017, https://english.stackexchange.com/questions/376024/origin-and-etymology-of-kush-cush-in-regards-to-animals.

p. 63   *In the United States it's "cush":* H. Carrington Bolton, "The Language

Used in Talking to Domestic Animals," *American Anthropologist* 10, no. 3 (1897): 75, 82, https://www.jstor.org/stable/658779?seq=18#metadata _info_tab_contents.

CHAPTER 14. CAMEL FEEL THE SOUL

p. 68   *among nonhuman mammals, they are second in intelligence only to dogs:* Animal Facts Encyclopedia, s.v. "Camel Facts," accessed July 9, 2019, https://www.animalfactsencyclopedia.com/Camel-facts.html.

p. 70   *By six they're considered mature:* Camel handler Doug Baum says that one camel year equals two and a half human years, but he's "not sure that any traditional camel cultures even ask questions like this and it's kind of a Western concept."

p. 70   *Female camels don't have a regular estrus cycle:* Hala Alfatlawy et al., "Overview of New Concepts in Induce Ovulation Triggers in Dromedary Camels," *ResearchGate*, June 2018, https://www .researchgate.net/publication/327655791_Overview_of_New _Concepts_in_Induce_Ovulation_Triggers_in_Dromedary_Camels.

CHAPTER 15. THE POWER OF CAMEL MILK

p. 73   *She's just done a double-blinded, randomized clinical trial:* Laila Y. Al-Ayadhi et al., "Camel Milk as a Potential Therapy as an Antioxidant in Autism Spectrum Disorder (ASD)," *Evidence-Based Complementary and Alternative Medicine*, August 29, 2013, https://www.hindawi.com /journals/ecam/2013/602834.

p. 74   *the often-valuable traits of honesty, dogged focus, intelligence, and pattern recognition:* Many people with ASD have skills that contribute to success later in life, but many more are too impaired by their condition to make full use of their talents. Although in tests people with ASD often display higher levels of intelligence and some kinds of cognitive skills than neurotypical individuals, very few are savants.

p. 75   *the composition of the microbiome:* Amy D. Proal, "Re-framing the Theory of Autoimmunity in the Era of the Microbiome: Persistent Pathogens, Autoantibodies, and Molecular Mimicry," *Discovery Medicine*, June 26, 2018, http://www.discoverymedicine.com/Amy-D -Proal/2018/06/autoimmunity-in-era-of-microbiome-persistent -pathogens-autoantibodies-molecular-mimicry.

p. 75   *It may be a factor in several diseases:* Like some forms of autism, some of these diseases have psychological components. See Michael Anft, "Understanding Inflammation," *Johns Hopkins Health Review* 3, no. 1

(spring/summer 2016), https://www.johnshopkinshealthreview.com/issues/spring-summer-2016/articles/understanding-inflammation. For instance, researchers have established links between rheumatoid arthritis and brain dysfunction. See Ana Sandoiu, "Rheumatoid Arthritis: How Chronic Inflammation Affects the Brain," *Medical News Today*, June 20, 2018, https://www.medicalnewstoday.com/articles/322207.php. Celiac sufferers are more likely to have traits of autism.

p. 75   *Pregnant women with inflammatory conditions:* Melinda Wenner Moyer, "How Pregnancy May Shape a Child's Autism," *Spectrum*, December 5, 2018, https://www.spectrumnews.org/features/deep-dive/pregnancy-may-shape-childs-autism.

p. 76   *Different types of autism are linked to gut bacteria:* Helen E. Vuong et al., "Emerging Roles for the Gut Microbiome in Autism Spectrum Disorder," *Biological Psychiatry* 81, no. 5 (Mar. 2017): 411–23, abstract available at https://www.ncbi.nlm.nih.gov/pmc/articles/PMC5285286.

p. 76   *A study of autistic children with gastrointestinal (GI) issues:* Destanie R. Rose et al., "Differential Immune Responses and Microbiota Profiles in Children with Autism Spectrum Disorders and Co-morbid Gastrointestinal Symptoms," *Brain, Behavior, and Immunity* 70 (May 2018), 354–68, https://www.sciencedirect.com/science/article/pii/S0889159118300783.

p. 76   *lactoperoxidase, found in all animal milk, tears, and saliva:* Zeynep Koksal et al., "An Important Milk Enzyme: Lactoperoxidase," IntechOpen, open-access chapter, September 7, 2016, https://www.intechopen.com/books/milk-proteins-from-structure-to-biological-properties-and-health-aspects/an-important-milk-enzyme-lactoperoxidase.

p. 76   *the enzyme NAGase:* Zafar Rasheed, "Medicinal Values of Bioactive Constituents of Camel Milk: A Concise Report," *International Journal of Health Sciences* 11, no. 5 (Nov.–Dec. 2017): 1–2, https://www.ncbi.nlm.nih.gov/pmc/articles/PMC5669503.

p. 76   *Lactoferrin can combat the growth of harmful gut microbes:* H. A. Almehdar et al., "Synergistic Killing of Pathogenic *Escherichia coli* Using Camel Lactoferrin from Different Saudi Camel Clans and Various Antibiotics," *The Protein Journal*, April 8, 2019, abstract available at https://www.ncbi.nlm.nih.gov/pubmed/30963371.

p. 76   *Children with autism-related immune-system deficits have a decreased ability:* Cecilia Giulivi, "Study Confirms Mitochondrial Deficits in Children with Autism," *UC Davis Health*, May 8, 2014, https://health.ucdavis.edu/publish/news/newsroom/8932.

p. 77   *The milk may also induce a calming effect:* Mohamed A. Hamzawy et al.,

"Leptin and Camel Milk Abate Oxidative Stress Status, Genotoxicity Induced in Valproic Acid Rat Model of Autism," *International Journal of Immunopathology and Pharmacology* 32 (Mar.–Dec. 2018), https:// journals.sagepub.com/doi/10.1177/2058738418785514.

p. 77   *GABA (gamma-aminobutyric acid):* A. Limon et al., "The Endogenous GABA Bioactivity of Camel, Bovine, Goat and Human Milks," *Food Chemistry* 145 (Feb. 2014): 481–87, abstract available at https://www .ncbi.nlm.nih.gov/pubmed/24128504.

p. 77   *nutrients that support the body's own population of beneficial bacteria:* Yuyu Shao et al., "Changes in the Nutrients of Camels' Milk Alter the Functional Features of the Intestine Microbiota," *Food and Function* 9, no. 12 (Dec. 2018): 6484–94, abstract available at https://www.ncbi .nlm.nih.gov/pubmed/30465678.

p. 77   *some children with autism lack several strains of beneficial gut bacteria:* "More Evidence That Autism Is Linked to Gut Bacteria," *The Economist*, May 30, 2019, https://www.economist.com/science-and -technology/2019/05/30/more-evidence-that-autism-is-linked-to-gut -bacteria.

p. 77   *The immunoglobulins produced by camels are tiny:* "How Camels Revolutionized the Antibody Engineering Industry," Twist Bioscience, December 12, 2017, https://twistbioscience.com/company/blog/how -camels-revolutionized-the-antibody-engineering-industry.

p. 78   *When digested, it can form beta-casomorphin-7:* Anna Cieślińska et al., "Treating Autism Spectrum Disorder with Gluten-Free and Casein- Free Diet: The Underlying Microbiota-Gut-Brain Axis Mechanisms," *HSOA Journal of Clinical Immunology and Immunotherapy* 3, no. 1 (2017), http://www.heraldopenaccess.us/fulltext/Clinical-Immunology-& -Immunotherapy/Treating-Autism-Spectrum-Disorder-with-Gluten -Free-and-Casein-Free-Diet-The-Underlying-Microbiota-Gut-Brain -Axis-Mechanisms.pdf.

CHAPTER 16. THE AMISH TAKE CAMELS ON FAITH

p. 89   *They're expanding in number:* Donald B. Kraybill et al., *The Amish* (Baltimore, MD: Johns Hopkins University Press, 2013).

CHAPTER 18. A FUNDAMENTAL EVOLUTION

p. 99   *"Autism Spectrum Disorder Treated with Camel Milk":* Christina Adams, "Patient Report: Autism Spectrum Disorder Treated with Camel Milk,"

November 1, 2013, *Global Advances in Health and Medicine* 2, no. 6 (Nov. 2013): 78–80, https://journals.sagepub.com/doi/10.7453/gahmj.2013.094.

p. 99   *When I go on a TV show to talk about the article:* Christina Adams, "Camel Milk to Treat Autism Symptoms," *Autism Live*, December 20, 2013, https://www.youtube.com/watch?v=ond93qHOsvg.

CHAPTER 21. CAMEL MILK IN THE NOBEL LAB

p. 121   *research that won the Nobel Prize in chemistry:* Felicity Barringer, "F. Sherwood Rowland, Cited Aerosols' Danger, Is Dead at 84," *New York Times*, March 12, 2012, https://www.nytimes.com/2012/03/13/science/earth/f-sherwood-rowland-84-dies-raised-alarm-over-aerosols.html.

p. 121   *"His body was making too much GHB":* "Succinic Semialdehyde Dehydrogenase Deficiency," NIH National Center for Advancing Translational Sciences, last updated February 25, 2013, https://rarediseases.info.nih.gov/diseases/7695/succinic-semialdehyde-dehydrogenase-deficiency.

CHAPTER 22. DOUG BAUM'S WORLD OF CAMELS

p. 130   *Doug's Texas desert treks:* Christina Adams, "Visiting with a Camel Up Close," author website, January 25, 2017, https://christinaadams author.com/visiting-with-a-camel-up-close.

CHAPTER 24. I AM A CAMEL BOY

p. 144   *"I trust what the Prophet (PBUH) said":* Devout Muslims add the parenthetical "PBUH" (peace be upon him) after invoking the name of the Prophet.

CHAPTER 26. CAMEL CLASHES AND CULTURES

p. 156   *"The culture was engaged in camels before Islam":* Eva Botkin-Kowacki, "History of Human Trade Is Written in Camel Genes," *Christian Science Monitor*, May 10, 2016, https://www.csmonitor.com/Science/2016/0510/History-of-human-trade-is-written-in-camel-genes.

p. 157   *"there were no camels in the Levant":* Mairav Zonszein, "Domesticated Camels Came to Israel in 930 B.C., Centuries Later Than Bible Says," *National Geographic*, February 10, 2014, https://news.national geographic.com/news/2014/02/140210-domesticated-camels-israel

-bible-archaeology-science; Elizabeth Dias, "The Mystery of the Bible's Phantom Camels," *Time*, February 11, 2014, http://time.com/6662 /the-mystery-of-the-bibles-phantom-camels; "Archeology Find: Camels in 'Bible' Are Literary Anachronisms," interview with Carol Meyers by Renee Montagne, *Morning Edition*, NPR, February 14, 2014, https://www.npr.org/2014/02/14/276782474/the-genesis-of-camels.

CHAPTER 28. INDIA REDISCOVERS ITS TREASURE

p. 165 *an article I wrote for* openDemocracy *about camel herders:* Christina Adams, "India's New Camel Legislation: Protection or Relegation?," openDemocracy, June 22, 2016, https://www.opendemocracy.net /5050/christina-adams/india-s-new-camel-legislation-protection-or -relegation.

p. 165 *Diabetes, now a major health concern in India:* R. P. Agrawal et al., "Zero Prevalence of Diabetes in Camel Milk Consuming Raica Community of North-West Rajasthan, India," *Diabetes Research and Clinical Practice* 76, no. 2 (May 2007): 290–96, abstract available at https://www.ncbi .nlm.nih.gov/pubmed/17098321.

p. 166 *camel milk reduced blood sugar levels:* R. P. Agrawal et al., "Effect of Camel Milk on Glycemic Control and Insulin Requirement in Patients with Type 1 Diabetes: 2-Years Randomized Controlled Trial," *European Journal of Clinical Nutrition* 65, no. 9 (Sept. 2011): 1048–52, https:// www.nature.com/articles/ejcn201198#subjects-and-methods.

CHAPTER 31. RAIKA VILLAGE

p. 189 *aak is used in Ayurvedic medicine:* Nanu R. Rathod et al., "Hypoglycemic Effect of *Calotropis gigantea* Linn. Leaves and Flowers in Streptozotocin-Induced Diabetic Rats," *Oman Medical Journal* 26, no. 2 (Mar. 2011): 104–8, http://www.omjournal.org/articleDetails.aspx?coType =1&aId=80.

CHAPTER 32. RAIKA COME IN FROM THE COLD (AND I COLLAPSE)

p. 191 *Camel Charisma, Ilse's nonprofit organization:* For more information, visit the Camel Charisma website at www.camelcharisma.com.

p. 199 *The valiant Raika herders:* For more information about the Raika, see the video "Autism (& Camel Milk) in India — Christina Adams," December 14, 2017, https://www.youtube.com/watch?v=AU3 GOf6tg80.

CHAPTER 33. LIFE IN "THE SAND"

p. 210   *it can even detect microbes that indicate the presence of water:* Paul Simons, "Camels Act on a Hump," *The Guardian*, March 5, 2003, https://www .theguardian.com/science/2003/mar/06/science.research.

AFTERWORD

p. 217   *Laws governing the sale of raw milk are changing:* Joanne Whitehead et al., "Recent Trends in Unpasteurized Fluid Milk Outbreaks, Legalization, and Consumption in the United States," *PLOS Currents*, September 13, 2018, http://currents.plos.org/outbreaks/index.html%3Fp=76143 .html?mc_cid=89c6279bf1&mc_eid=199646422c. Some countries outside the United States have specific health and safety challenges in camel milk production due to insufficient animal- and milk-testing infrastructure, vets, milking machines, chillers, and transportation.

p. 217   *Researchers are also exploring how the unique attributes of camels:* Alex Klarenbeek et al., "Camelid Ig V Genes Reveal Significant Human Homology Not Seen in Therapeutic Target Genes, Providing for a Powerful Therapeutic Antibody Platform," *mAbs* 7, no. 4 (2015): 693–706, https://www.tandfonline.com/doi/full/10.1080/19420862 .2015.1046648.

p. 217   *seasonal allergies:* "Camel Antibodies Provide Surprising Hope for Seasonal Allergy Sufferers," Medical Xpress, March 6, 2019, https://m .medicalxpress.com/news/2019-03-camel-antibodies-seasonal-allergy .html.

p. 217   *snakebite:* Sedigheh Khamehchian et al., "Study on Camel IgG Purification," *Human Vaccines & Immunotherapeutics* 10, no. 6 (2014), https://www.tandfonline.com/doi/full/10.4161/hv.28531; Jose Manuel Julve Parreño et al., "A Synthetic Biology Approach for Consistent Production of Plant-Made Recombinant Polyclonal Antibodies Against Snake Venom Toxins," *Plant Biotechnology Journal* 16, no. 3 (Mar. 2018): 727–36, https://onlinelibrary.wiley.com/doi/full/10.1111/pbi.12823.

p. 217   *sexually transmitted diseases:* Daria A. Burmistrova, "Genetic Passive Immunization with Adenoviral Vector Expressing Chimeric Nanobody-Fc Molecules as Therapy for Genital Infection Caused by *Mycoplasma hominis*," *PLOS ONE* 11, no. 3 (2016), https://journals .plos.org/plosone/article?id=10.1371/journal.pone.0150958.

p. 218   *But the very word* drug *came from the French:* A. N. M. Alamgir, "Drugs: Their Natural, Synthetic, and Biosynthetic Sources," *Therapeutic Use of*

Medicinal Plants and Their Extracts 1 (2017): 105–23, https://link
.springer.com/chapter/10.1007/978-3-319-63862-1_4.

p. 218 *people in the Boho Highlands:* "Bacteria Found in Ancient Irish Soil Halts
Growth of Superbugs — New Hope for Tackling Antibiotic Resistance,"
Phys.org, December 27, 2018, https://phys.org/news/2018-12
-bacteria-ancient-irish-soil-halts.html.

p. 218 *A report by environmental scientists at Yale University:* Jim Robbins,
"Native Knowledge: What Ecologists Are Learning from Indigenous
People," *Yale Environment 360*, April 26, 2018, https://e360.yale.edu
/features/native-knowledge-what-ecologists-are-learning-from
-indigenous-people.

p. 219 *these peoples live in regions that contain the majority of our planet's
biodiversity:* Claudia Sobrevila, "The Role of Indigenous People in
Biodiversity Conservation," The World Bank, May 2008, http://
documents.worldbank.org/curated/en/995271468177530126/pdf
/443000WP0BOX321onservation01PUBLIC1.pdf.

p. 219 *camels are the perfect animals:* Anas Sarwar Qureshi, "Fight Against
Desertification," *The Nation*, September 15, 2018, https://nation.com
.pk/15-Sep-2018/fight-against-desertification.

p. 219 *regions in Pakistan:* Asim Faraz and Abdul Waheed, *The Camel* (Beau
Bassin, Mauritius: Lambert Academic Publishing, 2019), 8.

p. 220 *pastoralism should no longer be perceived as "primitive":* "Partners Call
for Support Towards an International Year of Pastoralists," Food and
Agriculture Organization of the United Nations, accessed July 15, 2019,
http://www.fao.org/africa/news/detail-news/en/c/416207.

p. 220 *Milk and meat from pastoralists provide food security:* Personal interview
with Bernard Faye; see also "Pastoralism in the New Millennium," Food
and Agriculture Organization of the United Nations, accessed July 15,
2019, http://www.fao.org/3/y2647e/y2647e00.htm#toc.

p. 220 *satellite imagery is being used:* "Satellite Assisted Pastoral Resource
Management (SAPARM)," World Food Programme, https://www.wfp
.org/climate-change/initiatives/satellite-assisted-pastoral-resource
-management.

p. 220 *a study of children in northern Kenya:* For more on the health of settled
versus nomadic children, see M. A. Nathan, "Sedentism and Child
Health among Rendille Pastoralists of Northern Kenya," *Social Science
and Medicine* 43, no. 4 (Aug. 1996): 503–15, abstract available at https://
www.ncbi.nlm.nih.gov/pubmed/8844951.

RECOMMENDED READING

Abeiderrahmane, Nancy Jones. *Camel Cheese: Seemed Like a Good Idea*. Amazon Digital Services LLC, 2013.

Holton, Patricia. *Mother without a Mask: A Westerner's Story of Her Arab Family*. Dubai: Motivate Publishing, 2007.

Knoll, Eva-Maria, and Pamela Burger, eds. *Camels in Asia and North Africa: Interdisciplinary Perspectives on Their Past and Present Significance*. Vienna: Österreichische Akademie der Wissenschaften, 2012.

Köhler-Rollefson, Ilse. *Camel Karma: Twenty Years among India's Camel Nomads*. Chennai, India: Tranquebar, 2014.

Kraybill, Donald B., Karen M. Johnson-Weiner, and Steven M. Nolt. *The Amish*. Baltimore: Johns Hopkins University Press, 2013.

Tinson, Alex. *The Camel: The Animal of the Twenty-First Century*. Bikaner, India: Camel Publishing House, 2017.

INDEX

Aadvik Foods (India), 239
aak (edible leaf), 189
abandonment, 196
abattoirs, 201, 203
Abdi (author's Somali friend), 134,
    135–36, 137, 141, 145, 146, 147, 150
Abdul-Wahab, Walid: Amish farmers
    and, 94, 96–97, 152–53, 158; camel
    milk business of, 152–53, 159, 221, 237;
    camel milk business plans of, 91–95,
    97–99, 120; Facebook customer group
    of, 152; at Oasis Camel Clinic, 96–97;
    religious views of, 153, 158–59
Abeiderrahmane, Nancy, 227
Abraham (Biblical figure), 157
Abrahamic religions, 158
Abu Dhabi (UAE), 207. See also Al Ain
    (Abu Dhabi, UAE)
Adams, Jonah: autism symptoms of, 2, 4,
    5–6, 29, 36–37; autism treatment fail-
    ures with, 29–30, 38–39; current status
    of, 211–13; food sensitivities of, 6, 33,
    54–55, 78, 213; at mother's wedding,
    161; reaction to camel milk, 29–34,

35–37, 53, 54–55, 57–58, 112, 160–62;
    residence with father, 45, 54
adults, camel milk serving-size sugges-
    tions for, 230
Afghanistan, 201
Africa, 219
Africa, North, 156
Agrawal, R. P., 165–66
agribusiness, 220
Aisha (Mohammed's wife), 149
Al Ain (Abu Dhabi, UAE), 240; camel
    farm in, 205–9; camel souq in,
    200–204; oasis area in, 209–10
Al Ain Farms (Al Ain, UAE), 200, 205–9,
    240
allergies, 217. See also food sensitivities/
    intolerances
Amar, Sidi, 220
American Civil War, 129
Amish farmers, 60–62; as author's camel
    milk source, 56–58; camel milk sales
    of, 98; online activity of, 97; as pasto-
    ralists, 98; as undervalued, 219–20. See
    also Miller's Organic Farm

Amish farmers (*continued*)
    (Bird-in-Hand, PA); Troyer, Marlin;
    specific farmer
animal rights protests, 181
antibiotics, 181
anti-inflammatory medications, 181
antioxidants, 76–77, 121
A1 beta-casein, 78
April (camel), 214–16
Arab desert culture, 111
Arabian Peninsula, 157, 201
Ares, Mohamed, 148–49
arm contortions, 35–36
Artan, Ali, 137, 141, 142, 143, 146–48
arthritis, 71, 75, 90, 223, 231
Asperger's syndrome, 212
asthma, 75
attention, 34, 112
attention deficit disorder (ADD), 222
attention-deficit hyperactivity disorder
    (ADHD), 28, 66, 222
Austin (TX), 128
Australia, 18, 42, 71, 182, 211, 238–39
Australia Camel Milk NSW (Muswell-
    brook, NSW, Australia), 238
Australian Wild Camel Corporation, The
    (Harrisville, QLD, Australia), 238
autism spectrum disorder (ASD): in
    Amish community, 87–88; awareness
    events, 115; black children with, 74–75;
    bowel problems associated with, 79;
    cures for, 74, 120; dairy products and,
    6, 33, 122; factors influencing, 11; iden-
    tification "markers" for, 124; immune
    response and, 66, 75–76; inflammation
    and, 75–77; maturation time, 213;
    oxidative stress and, 73–74; rates of, 11,
    25, 53; symptoms of, 11. *See also* camel
    milk as autism treatment
autism conferences, 73–75, 83, 120

autism families, 67, 77, 166, 196
autism physicians, 38–39
"Autism Spectrum Disorder Treated with
    Camel Milk" (Adams), 99 ·
autism treatments, 213
Al-Ayadhi, Laila, 73–74

Babulal-ji (Raika camel herder), 177–78
bacteria, 125, 126
bacterial infections, 75
Bactrians, 41, 42, 68, 157
Bash (author's Pakistani acquaintance),
    7, 9
Baum, Doug, 128–33, 181
Bedouins: camel milk supplied by, 12,
    46, 57–58, 98, 106; as camel own-
    ers, 132–33; in Israel, 12, 42–43, 46;
    Mezzina tribe, 132–33; as Muslims, 106;
    Riegler and, 50–51; sedentarization of,
    43, 132; in Sinai Peninsula, 50–51, 128,
    131–33; Tarabin, 42–43, 46; in UAE,
    117, 210
behaviorism, 64
Ben (Amish farmer), 80, 84, 85–86, 88, 89
beta-casomorphin-7, 78
Bhopa (Raika wandering minstrels),
    192–93
Bikaner (India), 101, 102, 165, 194, 196
biodiversity, 219
biosecurity regulations, 228
Bird-in-Hand (PA), 80. *See also* Miller's
    Organic Farm (Bird-in-Hand, PA)
Birqash (Egypt), 133
black children, autism in, 75
Blake, Don, 121, 122, 123–24, 125–26
blood cells, 40–41
blood money, 142
bottle babies, 48, 64
bowel problems, 79
branding, 201, 207

brucellosis, 226
bull camels, 22–23, 49, 71
Bulliet, Richard, 155–59
bulls (cattle), 69
Burj Al Arab (Dubai, UAE), 115

Calamunnda Camel Farm (Kalamunda,
    WA, Australia), 238
California, 51, 134, 215, 237
Camelait (Al Ain, Abu Dhabi, UAE), 240
Camelait Camel Milk Asia (Shah Alam,
    Malaysia), 240
Cameland Negev Camel Ranch (Israel),
    239
camelback jewelry, 7, 8
camel boys, 141, 147–48
camel breeders, 48
Camel Charisma (Rajasthan, India),
    191–93, 194–97, 239
camel cheese, 191
camel clinics, 59–67
camel cultures, 68, 131, 170. *See also* Raika
    camel-herding caste (India); Somalia/
    Somalis
Cameleer India (online cameleer),
    100–104
cameleers, 56, 60, 90, 100–104
camel fairs, 42, 170, 180–85, 219
camel farms, 236–41; in Israel, 10; model,
    220–21; in UAE, 105, 107–11, 205–9.
    See also Amish farmers; Miller's Or-
    ganic Farm (Bird-in-Hand, PA); Oasis
    Camel Dairy (Ramona, CA)
camelids, 40–41
Camelicious (camel milk brand; Dubai,
    UAE): butcher shop at, 115; farm
    operations, 105–6, 107–11, 117, 119,
    240–41; gourmet products using, 220;
    processing plant, 114
camel markets, 200–204

camel meat, 113, 137, 148, 150, 164, 203–4
camel milk: allergic reactions to, 233;
    Amish, 56–58, 91; author's presenta-
    tions about, 66–67; cost of, 97–98; as
    dairy substitute, 5, 19, 78, 91; Facebook
    groups, 56–57, 60, 217; flavored, 108;
    gourmet products using, 112, 113, 114,
    145–46, 220; healing powers of, 2, 3, 4,
    12, 35, 66, 71, 76–78, 86, 124–25, 137,
    139, 146–47, 166, 222–23; Islam and,
    144; legality of, in Israel, 13; marketing
    possibilities, 79; nutritional properties
    of, 223–25; popularity of, 211, 217, 221;
    powdered, 205, 226, 228; price wars,
    152; production of, 12, 18–19, 22, 26,
    41; public sales of, in USA, 93, 98, 217;
    purchasing/handling suggestions,
    226–28; in Rajasthan, 189; raw vs.
    pasteurized, 91, 95, 105, 108, 123, 151,
    226, 231; sales of, in Rajasthan, 164–65,
    175; scientific research on, 5, 217–18;
    similarity to human breast milk, 3, 4,
    76, 121–22; solar-powered chillers for,
    183; in Somalia, 136–37, 142, 146–47,
    150; taste of, 91, 94–95, 108, 110, 129,
    226; transportation difficulties, 59, 154;
    usage suggestions, 229–32; where to
    buy, 236–41
camel milk as autism treatment, 222, 231,
    232–36; author's articles about, 59,
    99; author's interest in, 2, 4–5, 26–27;
    author's presentations about, 59, 65,
    66–67, 73–75, 112–13, 120, 165–68,
    196–97; author's procurement of, 9–17,
    28, 36, 37–38, 39, 45–46, 53, 56–58,
    59; cost of, 36, 46; disbelief in, 38–39,
    55–56, 75; dosages, 30, 35; Facebook
    groups, 56–57; FDA approval of,
    78–79; Jonah's reaction, 29–34, 35–37,
    53, 54–55, 57–58, 112, 160–62; popular

camel milk as autism treatment (*continued*)
interest in, 62, 79; raw vs. pasteurized,
105; scientific research on, 6, 73–74,
120–27; symptom improvement with,
34, 73–75, 112, 160–61; theories of, 35;
trials, 15, 28, 58, 73–74, 78–79, 114,
217–18; usage suggestions, 231, 232–36
Camel Milk Association (Branch, MI),
237
camel milk cheese, 114
camel milk chocolate, 220
Camel Milk Co., The (Kyabram, VIC,
Australia), 239
Camel Milk Co., The (Parker, CO), 237
Camel Milk Cooperative (Ridgefield,
CT), 237
"Camel Milk for Food Allergies in Children" (Yagil and Shabo), 6
camel milk lotions, 2, 25, 221
Camel Milk Smoothie recipe, 235
camel milk soap, 2, 23, 221
Camel Milk South Africa (Somerset West,
South Africa), 240
Camelot (camel), 21–22, 47–48
Camelot Camel Dairy, LLC (Wray, CO),
237
camel people. *See* cameleers
camel poop, 64
Camel Products (Netherlands), 240
camel racing, 42, 105, 117–18, 207
camels: basic needs of, 72; branding of,
201, 207; breeding, 65, 70–71, 110, 111,
133, 172, 192, 208–9; climate change
and, 219; colors of, 157–58; cows vs.,
217; diet of, 129, 131, 208; domestication of, 156–58; economic value of, in
Rajasthan, 164–65; feral, 182; horses
and, 50, 132; human uses of, 42–44;
importing of, 56, 66; intelligence of,
68, 72; mating of, 103–4; medical
testing of, 226–27, 236; memories of,
68; performing, 180–81; personali-
ties of, 68–72, 130; physiology of, 1,
40–42, 68–69; popularity of, 217, 221;
racing, 201; in Raika mythology, 192;
in religious history, 155–59; Riegler's
experience with, 50–52; sick, 181,
182–84, 194; slaughtering of, 201–2;
social dynamics of, 1, 42, 47–49, 65;
Somali songs/poems about, 138–39,
143; Somali view of, 134–35, 141–44,
146, 148–49; "spitting" of, 130, 181;
training of, 62–65, 70, 130, 221; types
of, 41; working, 64–65, 70, 133. *See also*
female camels; male camels
camel songs, 143
camel surgeons, 194
camel therapy, 26, 114, 206
camel tourism, 176–77, 181
camel urine, 138, 144
Camilk Dairy, 237
Camilk PTY LTD (Rochester, VIC,
Australia), 238
Canada, 51, 211
cancer, 144
caravans, 42
casein, 78
castration, 71, 182
cattle, 69, 156, 217
ceftriaxone, 181
celiac disease, 125
Central Veterinary Research Lab (Dubai,
UAE), 105
Chad, 42
Chapman University (Orange, CA),
18–19
cheese, 114, 213
chemotherapy side effects, 223, 230
Childhood Autism Rating Scale (CARS),
74

child murder, 196

children: with autism, introducing camel milk to, 232–36; camel milk serving-size suggestions for, 229–30

chloroform, 123, 126–27

Christianity, 158

climate change, 219

Clyde (Amish farmer), 57, 90

coliform, 126, 127

colitis, 75

Colorado, 79, 237–38

Colorado Camel Milk (Longmont, CO), 238

colostrum, 122

Columbia University (New York, NY), 155–59

Connecticut, 237

cow milk: allergic reactions to, 112, 122, 161; camel milk compared to, 77–78, 124, 125; donkey milk as substitute for, 161; elimination of, in diet, 167; Jonah's intolerance of, 6, 11, 33; nutritional properties of, 224–25; replacing with camel milk, 232–33, 236; transportation difficulties, 219; in UAE, 205; world-wide consumption of, 122

creationism, 97

Crohn's disease, 12, 35, 66, 75, 94, 222, 230

cushing, 63–64, 130

customs regulations, 228

Cyprus, 211

Dad, Mohamed Ali, 140, 141–49, 150

dairy products: allergic reactions to, 6, 54, 78, 112, 122, 213; autism and, 33; replacing with camel milk, 232–33, 236. *See also* cow milk

Dallas (Amish farmer), 57, 81, 90

Danaram-ji (Raika camel herder), 177

Daulet-Beket Farm (Aisha, Almaty, Ka-zakhstan), 239

Delhi (India), 177

Descartes, René, 156

Desert Farms UK and EU (UK), 241

Desert Farms USA (Santa Monica, CA), 237

diabetes, 86, 183; camel milk as treatment for, 125, 166, 195, 222, 230, 231–32; gas analysis and, 121; in India, 165; inflammation as factor in, 75; Raika community and, 165–66; scientific research on, 125

Diagnostic and Statistical Manual of Mental Disorders (DSM), 11

diarrhea, 94, 95, 147, 222

die-off response, 231

domestication, 156–58

donkey milk, 156, 161–62, 183

donkeys, 158, 162

dopamine, 77

Down syndrome, 166

dowries, 142

Dragon Slayers (Santa Cruz, CA), 51

Drome-Dairy (Watsontown, PA), 81, 238

Dromedairy Naturals USA (Centennial, CO), 237

dromedaries, 41, 68

drones, 219

Dubai (UAE), 200, 202; author's arrival in, 106–7; author's honeymoon in, 54; author's presentations in, 112–13, 115, 120; author's tourism in, 115–19; autism awareness event in, 115; autism therapy center in, 114–15; camel farms in, 105, 107–11, 241; camel milk/autism trials in, 105; camel milk products from, 145–46; camel races in, 117–18; heritage festival in, 116–17; souks in, 116, 118–19

Dubai Airport, 107

Dubai Creek, 116

Dubai Healthcare City (Dubai, UAE), 114–15

Dubai Mall (Dubai, UAE), 111–12

Dubai One TV (Dubai, UAE), 115

eczema, 75, 222

Egypt, 42, 128, 129, 131–33, 156, 239

Eid, 164

Emirates Airline, 106–7

Emirates Industries for Camel Milk Products (EICMP), 108, 240. *See also* Camelicious (camel milk brand; Dubai, UAE)

emotional speech, 34, 37, 112

empathy, 34

enzymes, 66, 76

eosinophil, 11

Ethiopia, 7, 144

"Etiology of Autism and Camel Milk as Therapy" (Yagil and Shabo), 6

European Union, 114

evolutionary theory, 97

executive functioning, 34, 213

Eyal (Israeli camel farm owner), 10, 12, 14, 16–17, 27, 28, 42, 46, 53

eye contact, 34

Facebook: Amish farmers using, 56–57, 60; author's cameleer friends on, 71, 91, 191; camel milk price wars on, 152; camel photos on, 64; Healing with Camel Milk group on, 56–57, 217; Healing with Donkey Milk group on, 162; Indian cameleers using, 100–104

falcons, 111–12

fatty acids, 76

Faye, Bernard, 220

female camels: milking of, 12, 22, 41, 84–85, 96, 110–11, 116–17, 206–7, 208; as mothers, 61, 65–66, 70–71, 214–16; pregnant, 48–49, 61, 70–71, 109–10; slaughtering of, 148; value of, 65–66

fine-motor improvements, 34

flocks, 42

food industry, 218

food sensitivities/intolerances: camel milk and mitigation of, 66, 74, 76, 222, 231, 232; to dairy products, 6, 54, 78, 112, 122, 213; donkey milk and, 161; Jonah's, 6, 33, 54–55, 78, 213; scientific research on, 6

France, 211

free radicals, 121

GABA (gamma-aminobutyric acid), 77

Gahlot, T. K., 194, 195

Gaj Singh II, Maharajah of Jodhpur, 192, 198–99

Gargus, Jay, 120–21, 124–26

gastrointestinal disorders, 76, 222, 231

Germany, 211, 239

GHB (gamma hydroxybutyrate), 121

goat milk, 6, 224, 236

goats, 156

Goldie (camel), 22

Gonenne, Amnon, 9, 35, 53; author's correspondence with, 10–13, 14, 15–16, 18, 27, 36; author's meeting with, 99; educational background of, 10

"Got [Camel] Milk?" (Adams), 59, 83

Great Britain, 211

Greenland, 211

grimacing, 35–36

gut health, 76

hadith, 142, 144, 157

harm (*Zygophyllum qatarense*), 209

Harrods (London, England), 45

Haryana (India), 102, 103

Hashemites, 132

Hashimoto's thyroiditis, 222

Hawaii, 60

Healing with Camel Milk (Facebook group), 56–57, 217

Healing with Donkey Milk (Facebook group), 162

helicopters, 219

Help in Suffering (nonprofit organization), 182

hepatitis, 66, 198

herd health certificates, 236

Hinduism, 164, 172

Hong Kong, 211

horses, 50, 132

Hostetler, Jeff, 238

Hostetler, Sam, 57, 61, 73, 81, 90, 122, 123, 238

human-animal connection, 156–57

human breast milk, 224

Humpback Dairy (Miller, MO), 81, 238

Hump Group (Birmingham, England, UK), 241

Hyderabad (India), 177

immune system, 11, 35, 66, 75–76, 231

immunoglobulins (IgGs), 77–78

India, 2, 211; author's honeymoon in, 54; camel milk sources in, 221, 239; "dryland" regions in, 219; hepatitis C outbreak in, 198; intercultural failures in, 172; online cameleers from, 100–104; Pakistan split from, 161. *See also* Pushkar Camel Fair (India); Raika camel-herding caste (India); Rajasthan (India); Sadri (India)

Indiana, 57, 79, 81, 90

indigenous peoples, 218–19

industrialization, 217–18, 219

inflammation, 11, 35, 75–77, 125, 181, 222–23, 230

insulin, 76, 166

intermarriage, 143

intermittent tic disorder, 231

investors, 62

Ireland, Northern, 218

irritable bowel disease, 14–15, 37, 94, 222

Islam, 43, 44; Bedouins and, 106; camels and, 156, 157; financial guidelines in, 159; gender-related customs in, 116, 139, 203; jihad in, 153, 158; Somalia and, 140, 142, 144, 149

Islam Question and Answer (website), 43

Israel: author's camel milk importation from, 7, 9–10, 12–13, 14–15, 106; Bedouins in, 43, 106, 133; camel milk legal status in, 13; camel milk sources in, 239; camel milk usage in, 94; modern, 10; Palestine and, 106; Riegler in, 27, 50–51

IUDs, 26

Jaipur (India), 163–64, 182, 186

Jaisalmer (India), 194

Jarisch-Herxheimer response, 231

Jeddah (Saudi Arabia), 92

jihad, 153, 158

Jordan, 132

Joseph (Biblical figure), 157

Judaism, 13, 157, 158

Juhász, Jutka, 105, 108–11, 113–15, 116–17, 119

Jumeira Beach Hotel (Dubai, UAE), 115

Kakar, Abdul Raziq, 68, 71, 200–207, 209–10

Kamelenmelk (Netherlands), 240

Kamelfarm Marquard (Hiddingen, Germany), 239

Kazakhstan, 18–19, 71, 239
kefir, 114, 122
Kenya, 7, 240
Khaleej Times, 113
kidney damage, 223
Kirsten (Camelicious PR rep), 105–6, 107, 113
Köhler-Rollefson, Ilse, 165, 166, 167, 174, 183, 191, 194–95, 199, 221
Koumama, Elhadji, 4, 7–8
Kumbhalgarh Camel Dairy (India), 221
Kuwait, 7, 211

laban, 114
lactoferrin, 76
lactoperoxidase, 76
lactose intolerance, 78
Lait de Chamelle (Risanni, Morocco), 240
language, 37, 112
lassi, 114
"leaky gut," 77, 78
Levant, 157
liver disease, 66, 223
London (England), 45
Los Angeles Airport, 36, 37, 45, 59, 98
Luna (camel), 65–66
lysozyme, 76

Maandeeq (Somali state camel), 134–35
Maasai people, 143
Machado-Joseph disease, 66, 223, 230, 232
Majlis Café (Dubai, UAE), 112–13
Al-Makhtoum, Mohammed bin Rashid, 106, 116
Malaysia, 240
male camels, 63, 69, 109, 129–30; bulls, 22–23, 49, 71, 208–9; control measures, 181–82; gelded, 71, 182; mating of, 71, 103; pregnant females and, 48–49; in Raika mythology, 192; sales of, in

Rajasthan, 175, 177; slaughtering of, 113; valuation of, 66, 113; working, 133
mange, 174, 181
mare's urine, 43–44
marriage, 142–43
Marwar Camel Festival (Sadri, India), 191–93, 194–97
matriarchy, 49
maturity, 213
Mauritania, 240
Media City (Dubai, UAE), 115
Mennonites, 61, 152
MERS (Middle Eastern respiratory syndrome), 226–27
Mexico, 71
Mezzina (Bedouin tribe), 132–33
micelles, 77–78
Michigan, 62, 79, 122, 123, 151, 214–16, 237
microbiome, 75
Middle East, 156, 219
milk: donkey, 156, 161–62, 183; goat, 6, 224, 236; mouse, 120, 124; nut, 6, 161; nutritional comparisons, 224–25; raw, sales of, 61–62, 91, 92–93; sheep, 187, 224; soy, 6, 161. *See also* camel milk; cow milk; *specific type*
Miller, Amos, 80, 81–84, 85, 94
Miller, Barbie, 87–88
Miller, John, 86, 89
Miller, Samuel, 80, 83, 84–85, 88
Miller's Organic Farm (Bird-in-Hand, PA): annual sales of, 83; author's visits to, 82–89, 94; camel milk operations at, 80, 83–85, 238; multifaceted operations at, 82–83
mind, theory of, 34
Missouri, 57, 61, 79, 81, 122–23, 238
Mohamedou (New York taxi driver), 155
Mohammed, Prophet, 149, 157

Moorpark College (Moorpark, CA), 23

Morocco, 211, 240

motor planning, 34

mouse milk, 120, 124

MRSA, 218

Mubarak (Al Ain Farms manager), 206, 207–9

Mudita Camels (Moffat, CO), 122

Mumbai (India), 163

mythology, 156, 172, 192

NAGase, 76

Nagy, Peter, 109, 113

Nashville Zoo (Nashville, TN), 132

National Institutes of Health (NIH), 124–25, 127

National Research Centre (Bikaner, India), 165, 194

natural therapies, 66

Negev Desert, 12, 42–43, 98

Netherlands, 211, 240

neurotransmitters, 77

Niger, 7–8, 98, 158, 220

Nobel Prize, 121, 126

nomads: American science and, 218; camel milk as sustenance for, 141; industrialization and, 219; lifestyle of, 150, 220; at Pushkar Camel Fair (India), 184–85; sedentarization of, 215; Somali, 143, 148–49, 150; as undervalued, 219–20. *See also* Bedouins; pastoralism; Raika camel-herding caste (India)

Northern Ireland, 218

nose pegs, 181–82

nursing mothers, camel milk for, 236

nut milks, 6, 161

Oasis Camel Dairy (Ramona, CA): author's visits to, 19, 20–27, 47–52; camel clinic hosted at, 59–67, 96–97, 128; as

camel milk business, 25–26, 220–21; founding of, 50–52; investors in, 25, 62

Oklahoma, 61

olive oil, 12

Oman, 201, 202, 205

Orange County (CA), 1

oxidative stress, 73–74, 76–77, 121, 124

Pabuji (Rajasthan folk deity), 172, 185, 192, 194, 195

Pakistan, 7, 160–61, 192, 200, 201, 211, 219

Palestine, 106

pancreatic function, 166

Parvati (Hindu deity), 172

Pashtun people, 204

pasteurization, 91, 95, 108, 123, 153–54, 226

pastoralism: advocacy for, 191; Amish farmers and, 98, 215; boundaries and, 215; camel as central to, 138; common elements of, 153; guests in, 142; Somalia and, 134, 138, 142; as undervalued, 219–20. *See also* Bedouins; nomads

Patrika (Indian newspaper), 166, 174

Peachey, Noah, 57, 61, 69, 80–81, 85, 97, 238

Pennsylvania, 57, 61, 79, 97, 238

peptides, 76, 78

pharmaceutical industry, 43–44

Philadelphia (PA), 80

Pichiyak (India), 186–90

pigs, 156

preeclampsia, 75

pregnancy, 48–49

Premarin, 43–44

price wars, 152

probiotics, 77, 114

Project K (university business plan project), 18–19

proteins, 76–77, 124

psoriasis, 222
PubMed, 5, 6, 56
Pushkar Camel Fair (India), 42, 170,
    180–85, 191, 219

Q Camel Dairy (Glasshouse Mountains,
    QLD, Australia), 238
Qur'an, 40, 43, 44, 157, 221

Rahmo (Abdi's wife), 135
Raika, Bhanwarlal, 193–94
Raika, Magan, 191, 193, 197, 221
Raika, Netha, 170–76, 177–79, 182, 183,
    186–89
Raika camel-herding caste (India): as
    camel-centric culture, 170, 172; camel
    economics among, 173–76, 177–78,
    195–96, 199, 221; camel milk consump-
    tion among, 165, 172, 189; cuisine of,
    173, 187–88; diabetes unknown among,
    165–66; industrialization and, 219; male
    camel control measures of, 181–82;
    oral tradition of, 174; at Sadri camel
    festival, 191–92; village life of, 186–90;
    youth and traditions of, 220
rain, 84
Rajasthan (India): author's presentations
    in, 165–68, 195–97; autism in, 168–69;
    camel as state animal of, 164; camel
    economics in, 164–65, 173–76, 177–78,
    195–96, 199; camel fairs in, 170,
    180–85; camel milk panel discussion
    in, 165–68; camel tourism in, 176–77;
    cuisine of, 173, 187–88; highways in,
    186; Raika village life in, 186–90. *See
    also* Raika camel-herding caste (India);
    Sadri (India)
Rajasthan Patrika media group, 165
Ramadan, 92, 93, 95, 164, 203–4

Ramona (CA), 20. *See also* Oasis Camel
    Dairy (Ramona, CA)
recipe, 235
response time, 231
rheumatoid arthritis, 75, 90, 223, 230, 231
rice milk, 6
Richard (camel), 129–30
Riegler, Gil, 20, 59, 90; Abdi and, 134; as
    author's Oasis Camel Dairy guide, 19,
    21–27, 47–48, 49–52; camel births and,
    66; on camel necessities, 72; on camel
    social structure, 48; camel-training
    method of, 63–64; career background
    of, 50–52; Israeli origins of, 27, 50–51;
    Israel visit of, 46
Riegler, Nancy, 23–27, 46, 59, 66, 90
robots, as camel jockeys, 117–18
Romeo (camel), 22–23
Rotana Hotel (Dubai, UAE), 107, 111
Rowland, Sherry, 126
Rub' al Khali (Empty Quarter), 201, 210

Sadri (India), 174; author's illness in,
    197–99; camel herders in, 193–94; Mar-
    war Camel Festival in, 191–93, 194–97
safari parks, 215
safety considerations, 226–27, 236
Sahara (camel), 52
Sahara Dairy Company (Newport Beach,
    CA), 237
Samatar, Salad, 146–47, 148, 149–50
San Diego (CA), 134
Santa Cruz (CA), 51
Saudi Arabia, 7, 91, 132, 144, 147, 153,
    158–59, 201, 211
sensory dysfunction, 223
serotonin, 77
serving suggestions, 229–31
Shabo, Yosef, 6
She-Camel (Patna, Bihar, India), 239

sheep, 178, 187, 188–89

sheep milk, 187, 224

Shiva (Hindu deity), 172

Sinai Peninsula, 42, 50, 131–33, 157

Singh Rathore, Hanwant, 165, 191, 192

skin conditions, 112, 222

sleep, improvements in, 112

sleep interruptions, 233

Smoothie, Camel Milk, 235

socialization, 65

social media, 90. *See also* Facebook

Somalia/Somalis: about (overview),
    140; autism rates in US community,
    135; camel boys in, 141, 147–48; as
    camel-centric culture, 134–35, 138–39,
    141–44, 146; camel milk as viewed in,
    137, 139, 141, 142, 146–47, 150; expat
    workers from, in UAE, 201; female
    camel herder from, 134, 136–39; Islam
    and, 140, 142, 144, 149; nomadic life in,
    148–49, 150; San Diego community,
    134

Somali Festival (San Diego, CA), 135

South Africa, 240

South Sudan, 143

soy milk, 6, 161

Spiers LTD (Nairobi, Kenya), 240

Stalzer, Meghan, 122, 123

stools, loose, 222

storage guidelines, 227–28

Studio One (Dubai TV show), 115

Sudan, 143

Sudani people, 204

sugar sensitivity, 222

suicide, 196

Summerland Camels (Harrisville, QLD,
    Australia), 238

superbugs, 218

Swami, Abhinav, 182–84

Tanzania (camel), 214

al-Tarabin, 42–43, 46

taurine, 120, 124

Tel Aviv (Israel), 10

Texas, 127, 128–31

therapy, 29–30

Thiaw, Ibrahim, 220

thrush, 223

Thulasiram, Chinnakonda, 114

Tibary, Ahmed, 65

Tiviski Camel Dairy (Nouakchott, Mau-
    ritania), 227, 240

Tony (author's husband), 91, 92; author's
    camel milk supply and, 45–46; author's
    marriage to, 54, 161; author's relation-
    ship with, 28–29, 54; British origins
    of, 45; camel milk consumption of,
    93; camel reactions to, 208; career
    background of, 28–29; children of,
    56; in India, 168–69, 176, 196, 197–98;
    Jonah's relationship with, 29–33, 212;
    in Philadelphia, 80; in UAE, 113, 114,
    115–16, 205, 206, 208

Torah, 157

travel considerations, 228

Troyer, Marlin, 197; as Amish camel
    farmer, 57, 61–62; apprentices of, 122;
    author's first meeting with, 60–62; at
    autism conference, 73, 83; camel birth
    on farm of, 214–16; camel milk busi-
    ness of, 151, 152–53, 237; camel milk of,
    126–27; conservative political views
    of, 92, 151–52, 215; family background
    of, 96; Miller brothers and, 82; at Oasis
    Camel Clinic, 96–97; online pres-
    ence of, 56–57, 60, 90; pasteurization
    opposed by, 153–54; safari park plan
    of, 215; Saudi students and, 92, 96–97,
    152–53, 158

Troyer, Savannah, 96

Tuareg people, 7–8, 56, 98, 220
tuberculosis, 66, 195, 226
Tunisia, 129
Turkey, 129, 156
turkeys, 48, 52

Udaipur (India), 194
United Arab Emirates, 2, 42, 54, 132,
    201, 211, 240–41. *See also* Al Ain (Abu
    Dhabi, UAE); Dubai (UAE)
United Kingdom, 241
United Nations Food and Agriculture
    Organization, 220
United Nations World Heritage sites, 201
United States, 51, 94; autism rates in, 11,
    25, 53, 135; camel clinics in, 59; camel
    milk and science in, 126; camel milk
    sales in, 93; camel milk sources in,
    237–38; customs regulations in, 16, 53,
    66; food industry influence in, 218; in-
    terstate milk sales in, 61–62, 91, 92–93,
    154, 217; male camel control measures
    in, 182; religion in, 158
United States Agriculture Department,
    37, 38, 39, 56, 66
United States Army Camel Corps, 128–29
United States Food and Drug Adminis-
    tration (FDA), 66, 78–79, 92, 153

University of California, Irvine, 6,
    120–27
University of Southern California, 96
Uttar Pradesh (India), 177

Valley Mills (TX), 128–31
Vergie (camel), 129
vet tests, 236
vitamins, 147
volatile organic compounds (VOCs), 121,
    124

weight gain, 112
White Gold Camel Milk (Nanyuki,
    Kenya), 240
Whole Foods, 98–99
World Autism Awareness Day, 115
World Bank, 219

Yagil, Reuven, 6
Yale University, 218–19
yeast, 167
yeast overgrowth, 223
Yemen, 201
yogurt, 114, 234
YouTube, 135–36

Zayed, Sheikh (UAE ruler), 205
Zygophyllum qatarense, 209

ABOUT THE AUTHOR

Christina Adams is the award-winning author of the memoir *A Real Boy* (Berkley/Penguin). She is a journalist and speaks internationally on writing, culture, health, autism, and camels. She has an MFA in creative writing from California State University, Long Beach. Her work has been featured by National Public Radio, the *Washington Post*, the *Los Angeles Times*, Gulf News, Dubai One, openDemocracy, OZY, WebMD, GOOD, Rajasthan Patrika, Tata Sky TV, Epocha, *Orange Coast Magazine*, *Global Advances in Health and Medicine*, literary magazines, and other publications. Her videos are viewed globally. In addition to writing, she's interested in style, regional food, history, and architecture. She lives in Orange County, California. Her website is www.christinaadamsauthor.com.

Twitter: @christinathink
twitter.com/christinathink

Instagram: @christina_adams_author
www.instagram.com/christina_adams_author

Facebook: @christinaadamsauthor
www.facebook.com/christinaadamsauthor